The Anti-Inflammatory Guidebook
© 2024 Future Publishing Limited

Future Books is an imprint of Future PLC
Quay House, The Ambury, Bath, BA1 1UA

A catalogue record for this book is
available from the British Library.

ISBN 978-1-80521-766-4 hardback

The paper holds full FSC certification
and accreditation.

Printed in Turkey by Ömür Printing, for Future PLC

**Interested in Foreign Rights to publish this title?
Email us at:**
licensing@futurenet.com

Editor
April Madden
Art Editor
Thomas Parrett
Contributors
**Edoardo Albert, Julie Bassett, Ben Gazur,
Bee Ginger, Madelene King, Jessica Leggett
and Alice Pattillo**

Senior Art Editor
Andy Downes

Head of Art & Design
Greg Whitaker

Editorial Director
Jon White

Managing Director
Grainne McKenna

Production Project Manager
Matthew Eglinton

Global Business Development Manager
Jennifer Smith

Head of Future International & Bookazines
Tim Mathers

Cover images
Getty Images

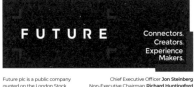

Future plc is a public company
quoted on the London Stock
Exchange
(symbol: FUTR)
www.futureplc.com

Chief Executive Officer **Jon Steinberg**
Non-Executive Chairman **Richard Huntingford**
Chief Financial Officer **Sharjeel Suleman**

Tel +44 (0)1225 442 244

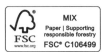

WELCOME TO

The
ANTI-INFLAMMATORY
Guidebook

Chronic inflammation, caused by illness, stress, injury or an autoimmune disorder, can sap your energy, leave you feeling unwell, and lead to further health problems. Happily there are ways to mitigate your risk of chronic inflammation, and even reduce it and its symptoms if you suffer from it already. From gentle and accessible lifestyle changes to delicious dietary swaps, we explain how you can take control of the causes of chronic inflammation and help you make a plan for positive change, so you can be healthier and happier for longer and reduce your chances of developing inflammation-related disorders. Let's get started!

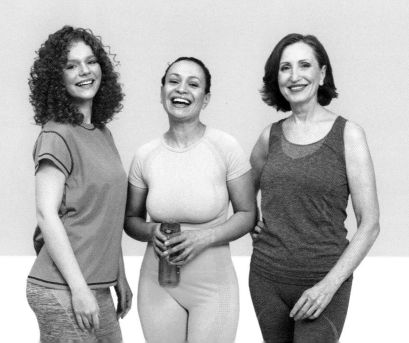

CONTENTS

1

SCIENCE

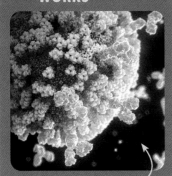

2

LIFESTYLE

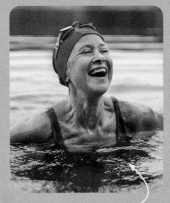

3

HEALTH

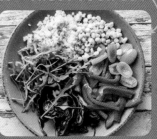

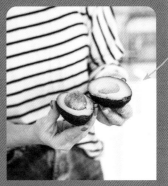

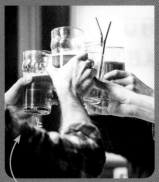

RECIPES

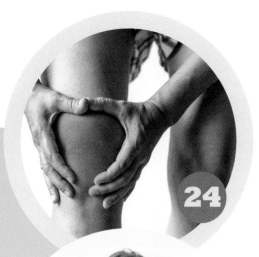

24

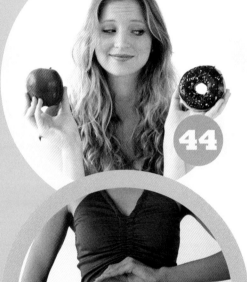

44

86

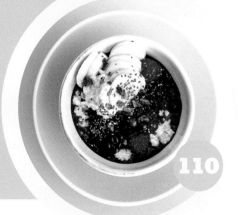

110

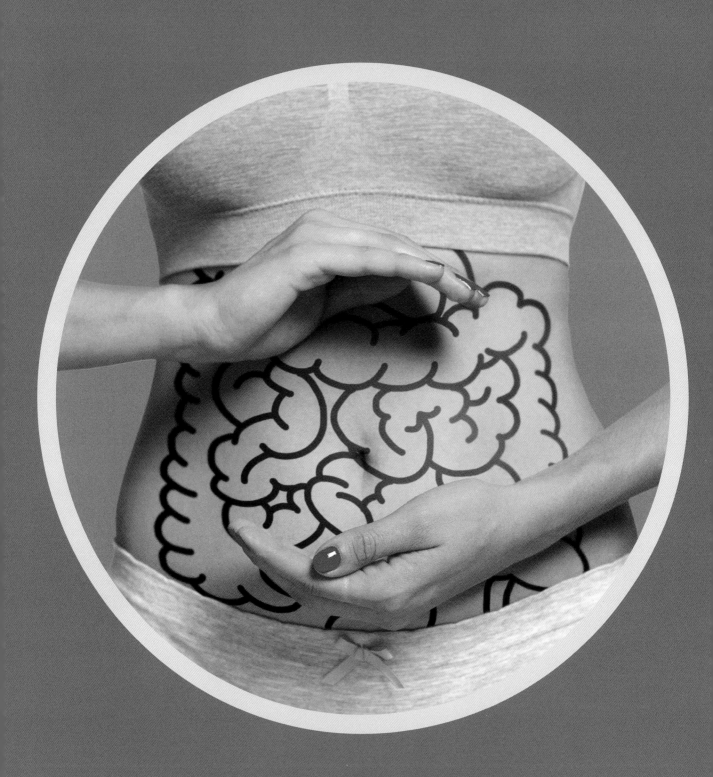

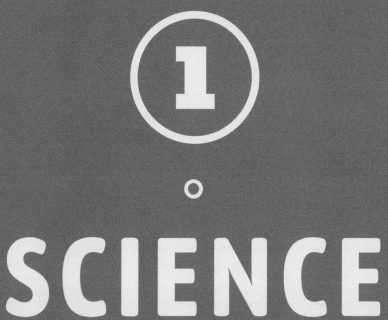

SCIENCE

///

Discover what inflammation is, how it works, and how to recognise its five key signs. Learn about its role in your immune response, and the disorders it can cause.

WHAT IS INFLAMMATION?

Inflammation is a natural part of our immune system. We explain what's happening inside our body, how it can affect us and when it can become a problem

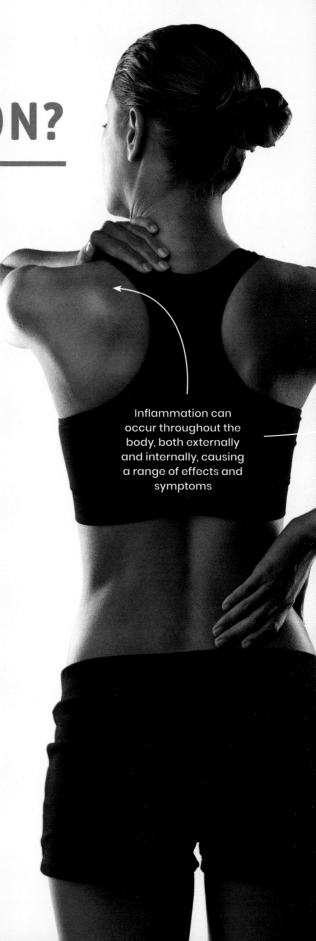

Inflammation can occur throughout the body, both externally and internally, causing a range of effects and symptoms

Inflammation is something that we will all have experienced many times in our lives. Which is a good thing, as inflammation is, under normal circumstances, a positive, natural reaction to trauma. It's part of our immune response, designed to protect and fight off damage to our body caused by an unwanted intrusion.

This type of responsive inflammation, which happens at the point of an injury or due to an infection, is necessary and required. However, inflammation that continues beyond the initial trigger is what can cause problems and symptoms over a longer period of time. Before we look at what this means and the difference between acute and chronic inflammation, it's important to understand exactly what is meant by inflammation.

The science bit

////////////////////

Inflammation kicks in when we're exposed to a virus or bacteria, chemicals or toxins, a cut or graze on the skin, an injury, or an external irritant, such as radiation or an allergen. When the brain detects a foreign object, an infection or an injury somewhere in the body, it signals certain cells to rush to help. These cells include white blood cells, inflammatory cells and a type of protein called cytokines.

The white blood cells and inflammatory cells are essentially the first line of defence, rushing in to fight off the detected intrusion. This might be to ward off any bacteria or viruses, or it might

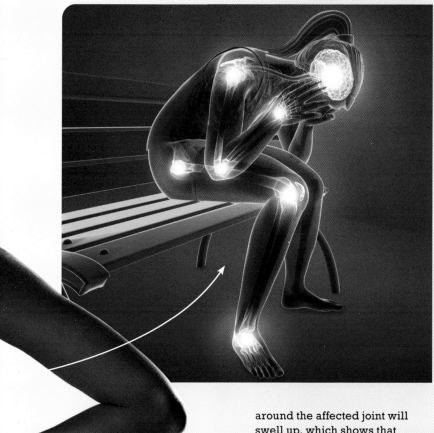

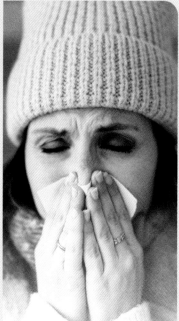

Something as simple as the common cold can trigger an inflammatory response, which is why you might get swollen tonsils or sinuses

be to protect damaged tissue if you've injured yourself. Cytokines are proteins that aid communication between different cells in the body and the immune system to form the right response to a problem. There are many different types of cytokines; some help the body to resist viral infection, while others help to direct immune cells to where they need to go. Cytokines help to regulate inflammation and control the body's immune response.

The effects of inflammation can be immediately obvious. For example, if you cut yourself, the area will go red, which is a sign that the immune system is sending extra cells to the area to prevent any bacteria from entering the body and prevent an infection. If you've twisted an ankle or wrist, then the area around the affected joint will swell up, which shows that inflammatory cells are getting to work by preventing further damage to the area and protecting the injured area. We explore the effects of inflammation, as well as the five key signs to watch out for, elsewhere in this book.

However, inflammation can happen internally where you can't see the effects. If you have a virus or have internal damage to an organ, these same processes will kick in. You may feel the effects, through tenderness or pain for example, but you won't visually be able to spot anything.

Acute vs chronic inflammation
/////////////////////

Inflammation, therefore, is a normal part of our body's processes and we need it. When everything is working as it should, your body's immune system will use inflammation to heal tissue or fight off an infection. The immune system should then know when to 'stand down' and trigger an anti-inflammatory response instead, to restore your body to normal. This is called 'acute inflammation', a normal and controlled reaction to trauma. We need this kind of inflammation, as it protects and heals our body.

Sometimes, however, the body continues to trigger and send out inflammatory cells even after the danger has passed, or when you don't need them, over a long period of time. This is what is called 'chronic inflammation', and is when it can become problematic. The excess immune cells can begin to attack the body's own healthy tissue and organs, causing long-term problems and a myriad of unpleasant symptoms.

Chronic inflammation can be caused by autoimmune disorders (where the immune system mistakes healthy tissue for unhealthy tissue and attacks it); exposure to external toxins (which could be due to a work environment or pollution); or untreated acute inflammation due to an injury or illness. We explore more on the known causes of inflammation elsewhere, though it's not always clear why someone suffers from chronic inflammation.

We're learning more about the long-term effects of chronic inflammation all the time. It is now being associated with many diseases, including Alzheimer's disease, cancer, heart disease and type 2 diabetes. The number of people suffering from some form of chronic inflammation and its effects is constantly increasing, particularly as the population ages.

It's important to know the difference between acute and chronic inflammation. When we talk about taking 'anti-inflammatory' measures that means looking to protect against or reduce the symptoms of chronic inflammation, not prevent the body's normal and desired inflammatory response to a valid trigger.

Common effects on the body

////////////////

Inflammation can occur anywhere in the body and for many different reasons. The effects can be quite varied, depending on where the inflammation is occurring and what kind of trauma has triggered the inflammation.

Think about the last time you had a common cold. Your body is working hard to fight the infection in lots of different ways, and this includes an inflammatory response. You'll often notice symptoms in your eyes, nose, ears or mouth, as these are the areas more prone to infection. You might get an earache, which is caused by inflammation of the ear canals in response to a virus. Your mouth is particularly vulnerable, which is why you might get ulcers on the lining of your mouth or inflamed, sore tonsils. Your sinuses may get inflamed, causing pain across your forehead and nose. In most cases, these kinds of symptoms are simply caused by the presence of a virus and they

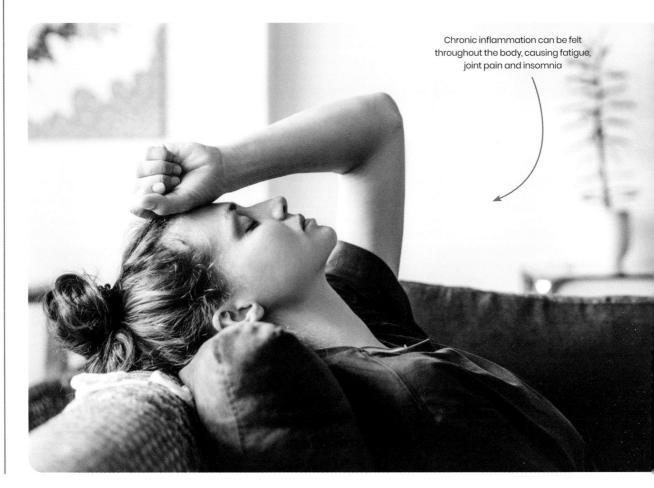

Chronic inflammation can be felt throughout the body, causing fatigue, joint pain and insomnia

"INFLAMMATION CAN OCCUR ANYWHERE IN THE BODY AND FOR MANY DIFFERENT REASONS"

will pass with time. However, if untreated, or if there are other stressors on the body (such as lack of sleep), then they may persist for a longer period of time. For example, chronic sinusitis is where the sinuses stay inflamed for three months or more.

Inflammation can also affect the body if you have allergies. You may notice a rash, swelling, blisters or redness in response

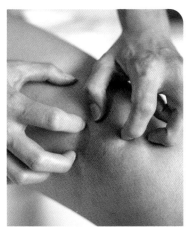

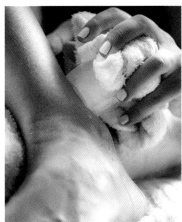

to a trigger. If you suffer from hayfever or other seasonal allergies, or react to pet hair or dust, then you might be familiar with the classic swollen red eyes or an inflammation on the inside of the nose (called allergic rhinitis). More serious allergies can cause rapid inflammation of the airwaves, which can prove dangerous and even fatal and requires immediate treatment.

The skin is quite prone to inflammation. If you cut yourself, you'll see redness and feel sore instantly, as the immune system jumps into action. There are also a number of inflammatory conditions of the skin, such as eczema, dermatitis and psoriasis, which can be chronic and may require long-term management and treatment.

Internally, any of your organs can suffer from the effects of inflammation. Asthma, for example, is the chronic inflammation of the breathing tubes leading down to your lungs, which make it harder to get a full breath in. Your heart can become inflamed too, which can lead to serious conditions such as arrhythmia (irregular heartbeat) and heart disease.

If you do have high levels of inflammation, regardless of whether it's short-term or long-term, this can affect you in other ways. You may feel more tired than usual as your body is working hard and you may also suffer from insomnia. You may have body pain, joint aches, changes to your weight,

digestive problems, changes to your mood or more frequent infections. This is where anti-inflammatory measures can make an difference.

Risk factors for inflammation

////////////////////

Any of us can be at risk of chronic inflammation, but there are some people who might be at an increased risk – for example, when lifestyle or environmental conditions can impact the body's inflammatory response.

Those who work in industries where they're exposed to chemicals, pollution or irritants on a regular basis may be more prone to long-term inflammation problems as the body is constantly trying to counteract the effect of these toxins without a chance to heal in between. The same is true of those who smoke, use drugs recreationally or drink heavily, as the body is continuously trying to battle the toxins entering the body.

People with some underlying and existing health conditions may also be more at risk of the effects of chronic inflammation. This includes those with diabetes (inflammation may be a contributory factor for type 2, but both types 1 and 2 can also be a risk factor for chronic inflammation). Our weight can also be a factor in our inflammatory response; some studies have discovered a link between an excess of fat cells and the overproduction of inflammatory cells.

Hopefully we've given you a good insight into what inflammation is, and some of the most common ways that it can affect the body, both positively and negatively to help you understand the importance of managing inflammation.

HOW YOUR IMMUNE SYSTEM WORKS

Your body is constantly primed to challenge the health threats that attack you every day

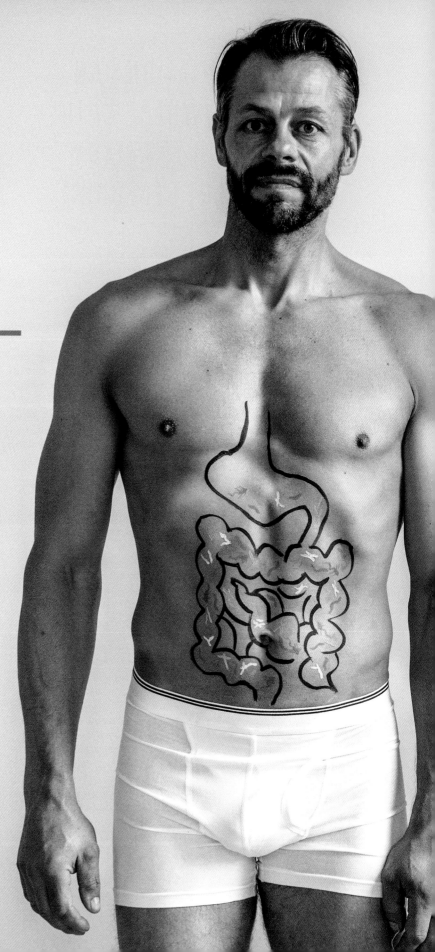

It's true: while you're simply sitting around watching TV, trillions and trillions of foreign invaders are launching a full scale assault on the trillions of cells that constitute 'you'. Collectively known as pathogens, these attackers include bacteria, single-celled creatures that live to eat and reproduce; protists, larger single-cell organisms; viruses, packets of genetic information that take over host cells and replicate inside them; and fungi, a type of plant life.

Bacteria and viruses are by far the very worst offenders. Dangerous bacteria release toxins in the body that cause diseases such as E. coli, anthrax, and the black plague. The cell damage from viruses causes measles, the flu and the common cold, among numerous other diseases.

Just about everything in our environment is teeming with these microscopic intruders,

"THE CHIEF NON-SPECIFIC DEFENCE IS KNOWN AS INFLAMMATION"

including you. The bacteria in your stomach alone outnumber all the cells in your body, ten-to-one. Yet, your microscopic soldiers usually win against pathogens, through a combination of sturdy barriers, brute force, and superior battlefield intelligence, which is collectively known as your immune system.

Physical defences

///////////////////////////

Human anatomy subscribes to the notion that good fences make good neighbours. Your skin, made up of tightly packed cells and an antibacterial oil coating, keeps most pathogens from ever setting foot in your body. Your body's openings are well-fortified too. Pathogens that you inhale face a wall of mucus-covered membranes in your respiratory tract, optimised to trap germs. Pathogens that you digest end up soaking in a bath of potent stomach acid. Tears flush pathogens out of your eyes, dousing bacteria with a harsh enzyme for good measure.

Non-specific defences

///////////////

As good as your physical defence system is, pathogens do creep past it regularly. Your body initially responds with counterattacks known as non-specific defences, so named because they don't target a specific type of pathogen.

After a breach – bacteria rushing in through a cut, for example – cells release chemicals called inflammatory mediators. This triggers the chief non-specific defence, known as inflammation. Within minutes of a breach, your blood vessels dilate, allowing blood and other fluid to flow into the tissue around the cut.

The rush of fluid in inflammation carries various types of white blood cells, which get to work destroying intruders. The biggest and toughest of the bunch are macrophages, white blood cells with an insatiable appetite for foreign particles. When a macrophage detects a bacterium's telltale chemical trail, it grabs the intruder, engulfs it, takes it apart with chemical enzymes, and spits out the indigestible parts. A single macrophage can swallow up about 100 bacteria before its own digestive chemicals destroy it from within.

Know your enemy: Bacteria

//////////

Bacteria are the smallest and, by far, the most populous form of life on Earth. Right now, there are trillions of the single-celled creatures crawling on and in you. In fact, they constitute about four pounds of your total body weight. Their anatomy is below.

The adaptive immune system

//////////////////////

When a pathogen is tough, wily, or numerous enough to survive various non-specific defences, it's down to the incredibly adaptive immune system to clean up the mess. The key forces in the adaptive immune

system are white blood cells which are called lymphocytes. Unlike their macrophage cousins, these lymphocytes are engineered to attack only one specific type of pathogen. There are two types of lymphocytes: B-cells and T-cells.

These cells join the action when macrophages pass along information about the invading pathogen, through chemical messages called interleukins. After engulfing a pathogen, a macrophage communicates details about the pathogen's antigens – telltale molecules that actually characterise particular pathogens. Based on this information, the immune system identifies specific B-cells and T-cells equipped to recognise and battle the pathogen. Once they are successfully identified, these cells rapidly reproduce, assembling an army of cells that are equipped to take down the attacker.

The B-cells flood your body with antibodies, molecules that either disarm a specific pathogen

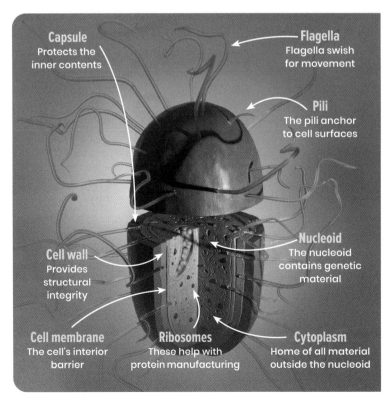

Capsule
Protects the inner contents

Flagella
Flagella swish for movement

Pili
The pili anchor to cell surfaces

Cell wall
Provides structural integrity

Nucleoid
The nucleoid contains genetic material

Cell membrane
The cell's interior barrier

Ribosomes
These help with protein manufacturing

Cytoplasm
Home of all material outside the nucleoid

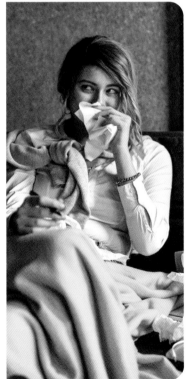

HOW B-CELLS ATTACK

B-CELLS TARGET AND DESTROY SPECIFIC BACTERIA AND INVADERS

① Bacterium
Any bacteria that enter your body have characteristic antigens on their surface

② Bacterium antigen
These distinctive molecules allow your immune system to recognise that the bacterium is something other than a body cell

③ Macrophage
These white blood cells engulf and digest any pathogens they come across

④ Engulfed bacterium
During the initial inflammation reaction, a macrophage engulfs the bacterium

⑤ Presented bacterium antigen
After engulfing the bacterium, the macrophage presents the bacterium's distinctive antigens, communicating the presence of the specific pathogen to B-cells

⑦ Non-matching B-cells
Other B-cells, engineered to attack other pathogens, don't recognise the antigen

⑥ Matching B-cell
The specific B-cell that recognises the antigen, and can help defeat the pathogen, receives the message

⑧ Plasma cell
The matching B-cell replicates itself, creating many plasma cells to combat all the bacteria of this type in the body

⑨ Memory cell
The matching B-cell also replicates to produce memory cells, which will rapidly produce copies of itself if the specific bacteria ever returns

⑩ Antibodies
The plasma cells release antibodies, which disable the bacteria by latching on to their antigens. The antibodies also mark the bacteria for destruction

⑪ Phagocyte
White blood cells called phagocytes recognise the antibody marker, engulf the bacteria, and digest them

THE LYMPHATIC SYSTEM

The lymphatic system is a network of organs and vessels that collects lymph – fluid that has drained from the bloodstream into bodily tissues – and returns it to your bloodstream. It also plays a key role in your immune system, filtering pathogens from lymph and providing a home-base for disease-fighting lymphocytes.

❶ Tonsils
Lymphoid tissue loaded with lymphocytes, which attack bacteria that get into the body through your nose or mouth

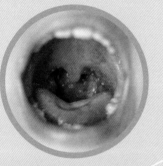

❷ Left subclavian vein
One of two large veins that serve as the re-entry point for lymph returning to the bloodstream

❸ Right lymphatic duct
Passageway leading from lymph vessels to the right subclavian vein

❹ Right subclavian vein
The second of the two subclavian veins, this one taking the opposite path to its twin

❺ Thymus gland
Organ that provides area for lymphocytes produced by bone marrow to mature into specialised T-cells

❻ Lymph vessels
Lymph collects in tiny capillaries, which expand into larger vessels. Skeletal muscles move lymph through these vessels, back into the bloodstream

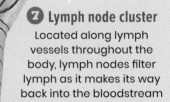

❼ Lymph node cluster
Located along lymph vessels throughout the body, lymph nodes filter lymph as it makes its way back into the bloodstream

❽ Left lymphatic duct
Passageway leading from lymph vessels to the left subclavian vein

❾ Spleen
An organ that houses white blood cells that attack pathogens in the body's bloodstream

❿ Thoracic duct
The largest lymph vessel in the body

⓫ Peyer's patch
Nodules of lymphoid tissue supporting white blood cells that battle pathogens in the intestinal tract

⓬ Bone marrow
The site of all white blood cell production

or bind to it, marking it as a target for other white blood cells. When T-cells find their target, they lock on and release toxic chemicals that will destroy it. T-cells are especially adept at destroying your body's cells that are infected with a dangerous virus.

This entire process takes several days to get going and may take even longer to conclude. All the while, the raging battle can make you feel terrible. Fortunately, the immune system is engineered to learn from the past. While your body is producing new B-cells and T-cells to fight the pathogens, it also produces memory cells – copies of the B-cells and T-cells, which stay in the system after the pathogen is defeated. The next time that pathogen shows up in your body, these memory cells help launch a counter-attack much more quickly. Your body can wipe out the invaders before any infection takes hold. In other words, you develop immunity.

Vaccines accomplish exactly the same thing as this by simply giving you just enough pathogen exposure for you to develop memory cells, but not enough to make you sick.

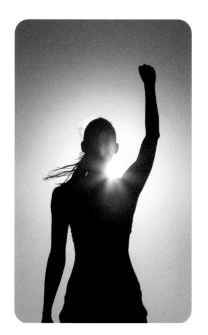

LYMPH NODES EXPLAINED

LYMPH NODES FILTER OUT PATHOGENS THROUGH YOUR LYMPH VESSELS

Your immune system depends on these .04-1-inch swellings to fight all manner of pathogens. As lymph makes its way through a network of fibres in the node, white blood cells filter it, destroying any pathogens they find.

1 Outgoing lymph vessel
The vessel that carries filtered lymph out of the lymph node

2 Valve
A structure that prevents lymph from flowing back into the lymph node

3 Vein
Passageway for blood leaving the lymph node

4 Artery
Supply of incoming blood for the lymph node

5 Reticular fibres
Divides the lymph node into individual cells

6 Capsule
The protective, shielding fibres that surround the lymph node

7 Sinus
A channel that slows the flow of lymph, giving macrophages the opportunity to destroy any detected pathogens

8 Incoming lymph vessel
A vessel that carries lymph into the lymph node

9 Lymphocyte
The T-cells, B-cells and natural killer cells that fight infection

10 Germinal centre
This is the site of lymphocyte multiplication and maturation

11 Macrophage
Large white blood cells that engulf and destroy any detected pathogens

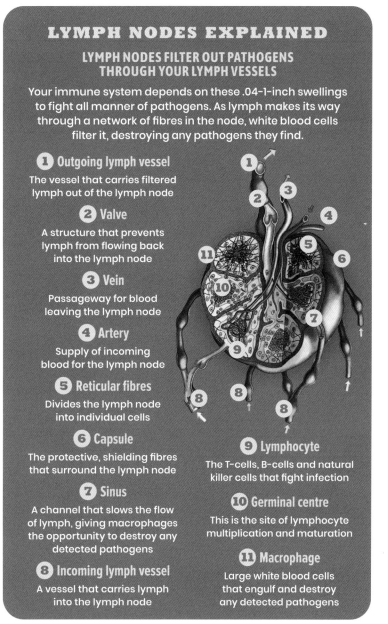

Disorders of the immune system
//////////////////////////

The immune system is a powerful set of defences, so when it malfunctions, it can do as much harm as a disease. Allergies are the result of an overzealous immune system. In response to something that is relatively benign, like pollen for example, the immune system will trigger excessive measures to expel the pathogen. In extreme cases, allergies cause anaphylactic shock, which is a potentially deadly drop in blood pressure, sometimes accompanied by breathing difficulty and loss of consciousness. In autoimmune disorders such as rheumatoid arthritis, the immune system fails to recognise the body's own cells and attacks them.

Images Getty, Ed Uthman; MD (lymphatic system close-up), DK Images (lymphatic system body)

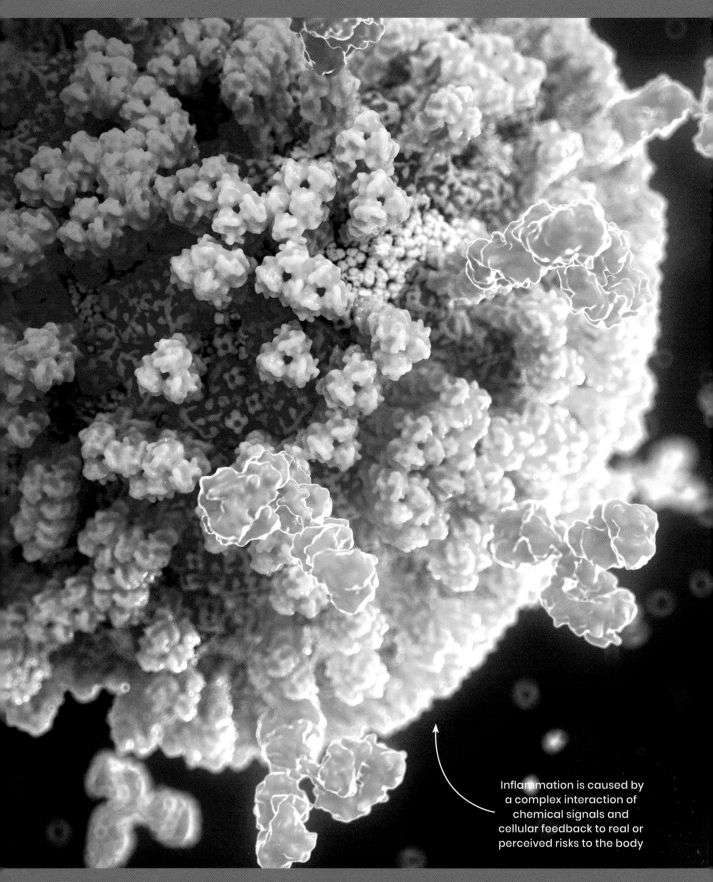

Inflammation is caused by a complex interaction of chemical signals and cellular feedback to real or perceived risks to the body

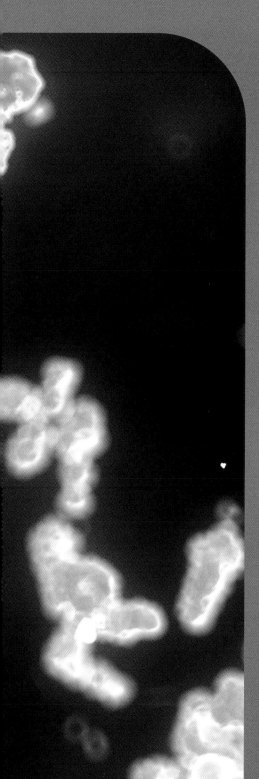

CAUSES OF INFLAMMATION

INFLAMMATION IS ONE OF OUR NATURAL DEFENSES, BUT WHAT TRIGGERS IT AND WHAT MAKES IT A SERIOUS CONDITION?

The human body is an exquisite machine capable of wonderful things. Over billions of years of evolution it has been refined into an intricate mechanism designed to keep us alive against the dangers of the world we live in. One of the most complex aspects of our bodies is the immune system that fights the bacteria, viruses, and other nasty foreign objects that surround us. Inflammation is the result of our immune systems preparing for a battle.

When the body detects damage or danger it springs into action. Imagine cut on your finger. To us it may seem like a minor injury but the body reacts instantly. Any break in the skin can let pathogen bacteria in. The first response of the body is to begin clotting to stop blood loss. The platelets responsible for this release a chemical signal known as cytokines which draws the other components of the immune system to the area. Specialist white blood cells, called neutrophils, arrive to envelop and digest any bacteria present as well as any damaged cells caused by the wound. It is the arrival of the chemicals and cells of the immune response which cause the symptoms of inflammation.

Obvious injuries like a cut are just one of the things which can trigger inflammation because there are numerous routes through which infection and contamination can enter the body. A bacterium anywhere in the blood stream must be dealt with, as must a virus. Anything that causes the immune response is known as an antigen. Antigens are often the proteins which are found on the exterior of a foreign cell as it is these proteins which allow the body to tell 'friend' from 'foe'. When these are detected by antibodies or white blood cells the immune response is turned on and inflammation is caused at the site. The immune system can also respond to proteins on our own cells which are misshapen or normally on the inside of a cell as this clears away damaged cells and potentially cancerous ones.

Non-living things can also cause the immune system to be activated. Toxins, dangerous chemicals, and medical implants can also sometimes be antigenic.

Because the immune system is so complex it sometimes makes an incorrect detection of danger. This is why some people develop allergies and intolerance for certain substances. Occasionally, the immune system will turn against the body's own cells and cause widespread inflammation in conditions known as autoimmune diseases.

"THE IMMUNE RESPONSE CAUSES THE SYMPTOMS OF INFLAMMATION"

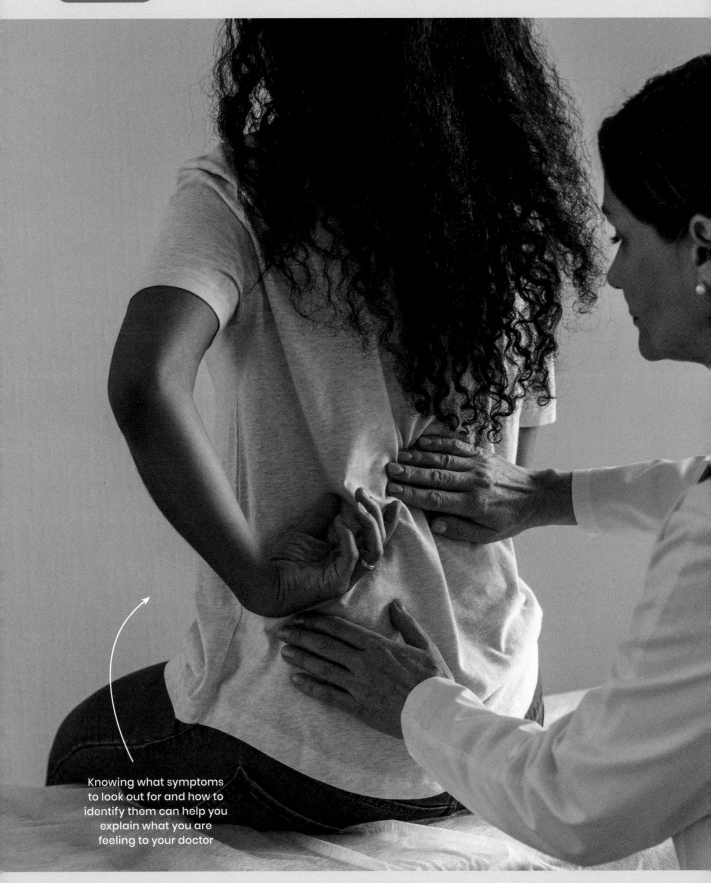

Knowing what symptoms to look out for and how to identify them can help you explain what you are feeling to your doctor

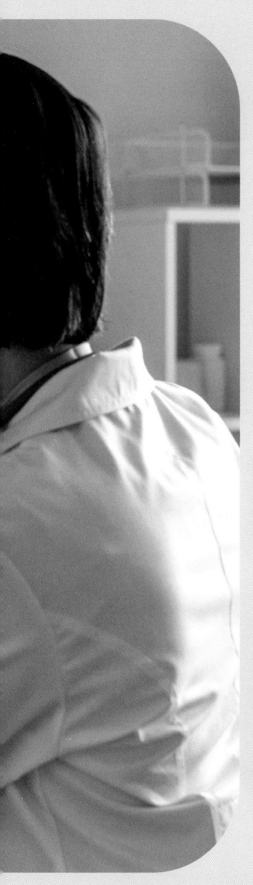

EFFECTS OF INFLAMMATION

While inflammation is a vital part of our bodies' ability to keep us safe it is not one which most people understand in detail. It has also recently been implicated in a wide range of illnesses which blight the lives of millions. From arthritis to heart disease to depression, the influence of inflammation is being investigated. But what signs and symptoms of inflammation should you look out for?

Acute inflammation, that which is caused by a clear cause, is relatively easy to spot. Inflammation is usually defined by five key symptoms: pain, heat, loss of function, redness, and swelling. Everyone will have experienced these after an injury or allergic response, and they usually disappear quite quickly.

To identify inflammation you can perform some simple checks. When you rest your hand on the area it might feel hot to the touch when compared to the flesh around it. Colour changes can be startling if it appears a vivid red but more subtle colour differences may also point to inflammation, especially in people of colour. Compare similar areas on your body to look for differences in hue. Swelling caused by inflammation will make the area feel hard or tight when you move it. To spot swelling it may be helpful to compare it to the same area on the other side of your body. For instance it is easier to spot swelling on a foot by placing it beside your other foot. It is swelling which causes the pain associated with inflammation. This can feel like a throbbing ache or a sharp stabbing sensation. It is due to both the pain and swelling that you may not be able to use the body part affected.

Chronic inflammation is a more tricky condition to spot than acute symptoms in many cases. The symptoms of inflammation may develop more slowly in a chronic condition and will last for a longer period, often with no obvious cause. The causes of chronic inflammation will need to be investigated by a doctor but there are clues you can look out for to help you identify it.

The symptoms may be systemic, meaning they effect the whole body. A fever can be a sign of chronic inflammation. You may have multiple pains in several joints. Suffering from rashes and itchy skin over wide areas could be a symptom. Long lasting gastrointestinal symptoms could also point towards suffering from a chronic inflammatory disease.

"CHRONIC INFLAMMATION IS A TRICKY CONDITION TO SPOT IN MANY CASES"

Image Getty

23

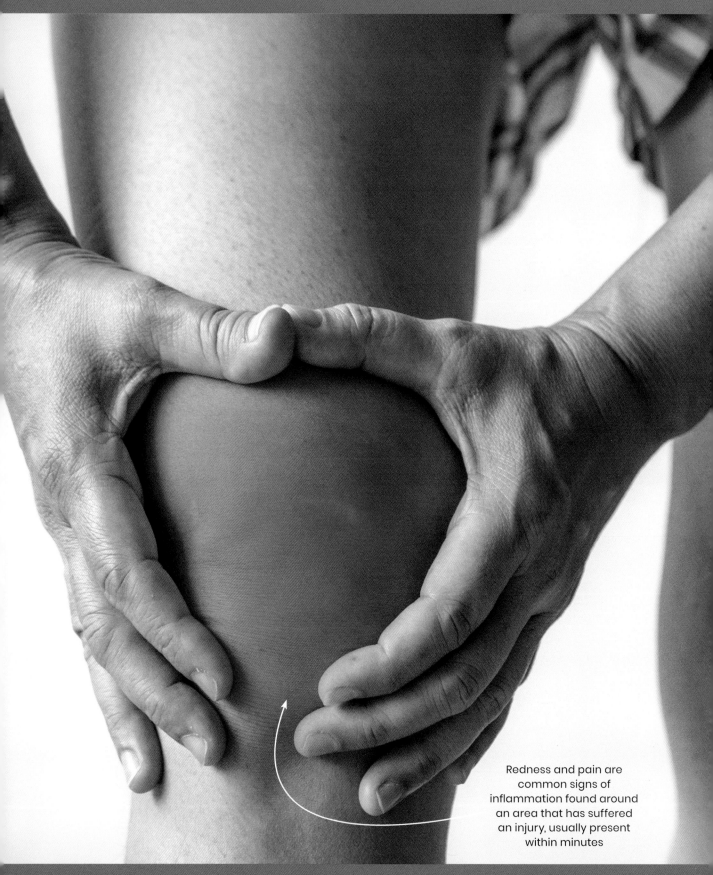

Redness and pain are common signs of inflammation found around an area that has suffered an injury, usually present within minutes

{ 5 KEY SIGNS OF INFLAMMATION }

DO YOU KNOW HOW TO RECOGNISE INFLAMMATION IN THE BODY? HERE ARE THE TOP INDICATORS TO WATCH OUT FOR AND WHY THEY HAPPEN

When your body is suffering from inflammation, whether due to infection, injury or illness, it will respond physically, indicating that something is wrong. These signals can help to identify or diagnose a problem… if you know what you're looking for. Here is our quick guide to the five key signs of inflammation.

❶ Redness

If you have a cut or injury, one of the things you might notice straight away is that the area goes red. This is a sign that the small blood vessels are dilating around the problem area, enabling more blood through to aid the healing process. The enhanced blood flow also carries extra immune system cells to prevent or fight infection, and to begin to repair damage.

❷ Swelling

If you've ever twisted your ankle, for example, you will have noticed that it swells up pretty fast. This swelling, called edema, is present in areas where fluid builds up. If it's close to the surface, you will be able to see the affected area swell, but it can happen internally throughout the body too. The excess fluid is due to the dilated blood vessels carrying more volume to one area, and leaking out into the surrounding cells.

❸ Heat

As the blood vessels dilate and blood flow increases, the inflamed area of the body can start to feel warm to the touch. This is usually isolated in the case of an injury or wound on the skin. If joints are inflamed, such as in the case of arthritis, these areas may also feel warm. If the body is fighting an infection or illness, then this can cause full-body fevers.

❹ Pain

Inflammation and pain go hand in hand. Parts of the body that are suffering from inflammation can be sensitive to touch or be painful to move. If there's swelling, this can push on the surrounding skin, causing increased pain. The immune system also releases hormones that signal pain – a protective response to stop us from moving the affected area.

❺ Loss of function

One of the more significant signs of inflammation is a loss of function in the affected area. This might mean that a joint is difficult or stiff to move, for example, while it's inflamed. If the inflammation is in or around an organ, it can prevent it from doing its job the way it should, for example it's hard to breathe properly when there's inflammation in the lungs.

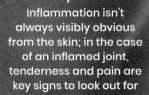

Inflammation isn't always visibly obvious from the skin; in the case of an inflamed joint, tenderness and pain are key signs to look out for

Image Getty

25

INFLAMMATION: ITS SIGNS AND SYMPTOMS

What are the symptoms of chronic inflammation and how is it diagnosed?

The body is designed to remain stable. Human beings have lived everywhere, from the tropics to the Arctic, but wherever we live, the conditions inside the body remain the same: the same temperature, the same fluid balance, the same blood pressure. When these conditions change – a high temperature, for instance – we know at once that something is wrong. But in the normal course of events, the body responds to changing conditions without us even noticing. This is known as homeostasis. It is the body's dynamic equilibrium with its environment. It is a dynamic rather than a static equilibrium because it is maintained by the body changing its response to the environment.

Stress and homeostasis

///////////////////////

Stress is by no means always bad. Indeed, quite the opposite: it is vital. Stress is the body's response to a need to change. The change can be something as simple as the sun going down. The temperature drops and the body prepares to go to sleep. It can be something as sudden and dramatic as hearing movement in the long grass and glimpsing tawny fur. Then it's all systems go as the body triggers its flight/fight reaction.

An emergency – spotting a hunting lion or the car skidding – triggers the body's emergency response system. This is known medically as acute stress and it's the response to sudden danger. The body responds to acute stress by firing up the autonomic nervous system, which comprises the sympathetic and parasympathetic nervous systems. The sympathetic nervous system (the flight/fight system) releases a range of neurotransmitters and hormones that increase the heart rate, as well as the blood flow to muscles, the brain, and to the senses. Meanwhile, the parasympathetic nervous system (descriptively called the rest/digest system) is closed down. We are ready for action. However, if we are in a situation that triggers this response but the situation does not quickly resolve itself – say the long-term stress of a gaslighting boss – then we are on course for developing hypertension, one of the main causes of chronic inflammation.

Acute stress also triggers the hypothalamus, a deep part of the brain, which then stimulates the pituitary gland, which in turn triggers the production of cortisol. Cortisol is the body's main stress hormone. As a hormone, it facilitates the production of energy and triggers the immune system. The sort of emergencies that we used to face often produced injuries. Cortisol mobilises the body to deal with this: the inflammation surrounding a wound is the body activating white blood cells to deal with pathogens. But when acute stress turns into chronic stress, and the cortisol levels remain consistently high, then the body is in danger of suffering from oxidative stress, leading to chronic inflammation.

Symptoms of chronic inflammation

///////////////////////

Chronic inflammation can affect particular systems and different parts of the body. It can also be generalised, operating at a low level throughout the body. So not surprisingly, the possible symptoms are quite varied. To give you an idea, they can include chronic fatigue, general or local body pain, recurring infections, diarrhoea, constipation, weight loss, weight gain, depression, anxiety, mood disorders and Alzheimer's.

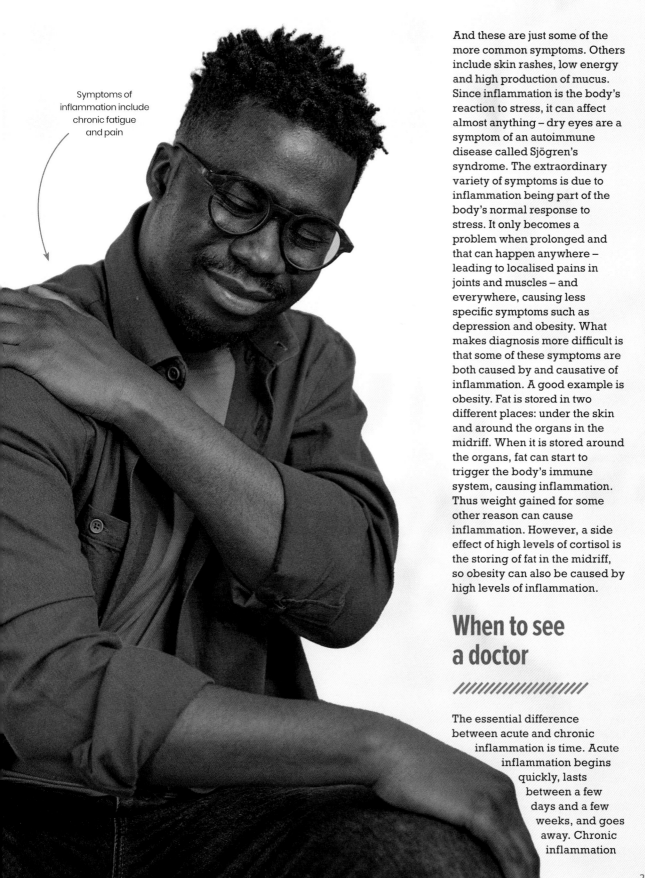

Symptoms of inflammation include chronic fatigue and pain

And these are just some of the more common symptoms. Others include skin rashes, low energy and high production of mucus. Since inflammation is the body's reaction to stress, it can affect almost anything – dry eyes are a symptom of an autoimmune disease called Sjögren's syndrome. The extraordinary variety of symptoms is due to inflammation being part of the body's normal response to stress. It only becomes a problem when prolonged and that can happen anywhere – leading to localised pains in joints and muscles – and everywhere, causing less specific symptoms such as depression and obesity. What makes diagnosis more difficult is that some of these symptoms are both caused by and causative of inflammation. A good example is obesity. Fat is stored in two different places: under the skin and around the organs in the midriff. When it is stored around the organs, fat can start to trigger the body's immune system, causing inflammation. Thus weight gained for some other reason can cause inflammation. However, a side effect of high levels of cortisol is the storing of fat in the midriff, so obesity can also be caused by high levels of inflammation.

When to see a doctor

/////////////////////

The essential difference between acute and chronic inflammation is time. Acute inflammation begins quickly, lasts between a few days and a few weeks, and goes away. Chronic inflammation

Images Getty

27

begins slowly, gradually worsening, and then lingers on, often indefinitely. Acute inflammation is usually connected to something definite: an injury, a disease or exposure to a toxin, or a particular shock, which helps to tie down its cause. Chronic inflammation is much more difficult to pin on anything specific as it is usually caused by the slow build-up of a number of different factors. So make an appointment to see a doctor if the condition is ongoing, shows no sign of improving, and has no obvious cause.

Diagnosing chronic inflammation

In diagnosing chronic inflammation, doctors will first look at the symptoms the patient is presenting and try to establish possible causes for these. But if, having considered alternative possibilities, chronic inflammation remains a possibility, the doctor will likely consider one of a number of tests to check for inflammatory markers in the system. Although these tests do not directly check for inflammation, they instead search for signs that the system is inflamed.

Among the tests to check for inflammation are:
Erythrocyte sedimentation rate (more snappily named sed rate or ESR). This tests how long it takes for red blood cells to settle to the bottom of a test tube. Inflammation makes the red blood cells settle quicker.

C-reactive protein (CRP). The levels of this protein usually rise in cases of chronic inflammation, rising from a normal level of 3mg/l to over 100mg/l.

Test for ferritin. This is a blood protein linked to iron levels in the body. The test is used to check for anaemia, when levels of ferritin will be very low, but high levels of the protein are likely to indicate possible inflammation.

Testing fibrinogen. This test checks how well the body's blood-clotting system is working, but again the level of the protein often rises in cases of chronic inflammation. None of the tests for inflammation confirm, on their own, the presence of chronic inflammation: a doctor will use them alongside other symptoms before making a diagnosis.

Diseases of chronic inflammation

As already mentioned, it is difficult to work out the causative links of the diseases associated with chronic inflammation. However, what is clear is that these diseases exacerbate inflammation,

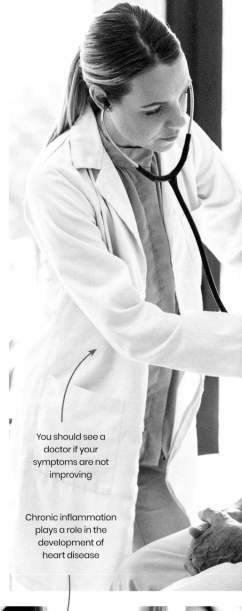

You should see a doctor if your symptoms are not improving

Chronic inflammation plays a role in the development of heart disease

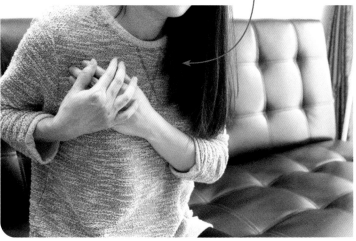

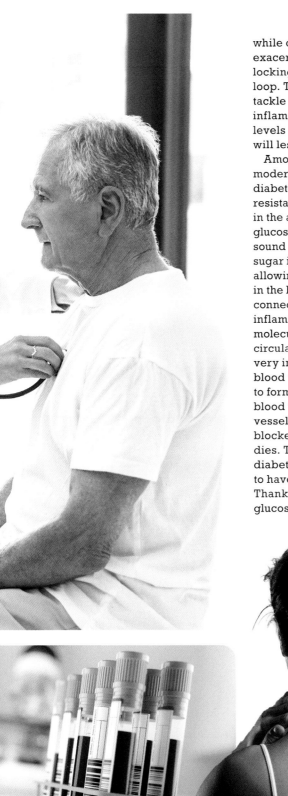

while chronic inflammation exacerbates the diseases, locking the body into a feedback loop. Therefore, helping to tackle the disease will ease the inflammation and reducing the levels of chronic inflammation will lessen the disease.

Among the most common of modern-day diseases is type-2 diabetes, which produces insulin resistance, leading to a reduction in the ability of cells to turn glucose into fat. This might not sound so bad – who wants to turn sugar into fat after all – but allowing glucose to float around in the bloodstream is where the connection with chronic inflammation comes in. Glucose molecules, when allowed to circulate in the bloodstream, are very inflammatory. They irritate blood vessels, causing plaques to form, which slowly block blood vessels. When blood vessels become completely blocked, the surrounding tissue dies. This is why people with diabetes can go blind and have to have limbs amputated. Thankfully, a diet cutting out glucose and effective weight loss can stop and even reverse type-2 diabetes, making it one of the disorders amenable to the patient helping themselves.

Heart disease is the major cause of death for men in the UK and is high on the list of causes of death in women. In the public mind, it's not a disease commonly associated with chronic inflammation but inflammation plays a crucial role in the disease's development. As with diabetes, heart disease results from plaques forming in the blood vessels around the heart. These plaques are often the result of the interior lining of the blood vessels becoming inflamed. Thus reducing inflammation in and around the heart reduces the risk of a heart attack. Statins are prescribed to reduce the build up of plaque in and around the heart and research shows that these are very effective drugs. However, research also indicates that making the switch to a low-inflammatory diet will reduce the inflammation markers around the heart, and help reduce the risk of a heart attack.

All the diseases associated with chronic inflammation follow the normal pattern of chronic diseases: being slow to develop and long-lasting. As such, they are strong evidence for the advantages in taking up a low-inflammation diet and lifestyle. Doing so will reduce or curtail many of the factors leading to chronic inflammation, and thus remove many of the diseases that, in the modern world, plague the last years of so many peoples' lives. No one lives forever but it is possible to live well until the end if we make the right sorts of choices today and from here on in.

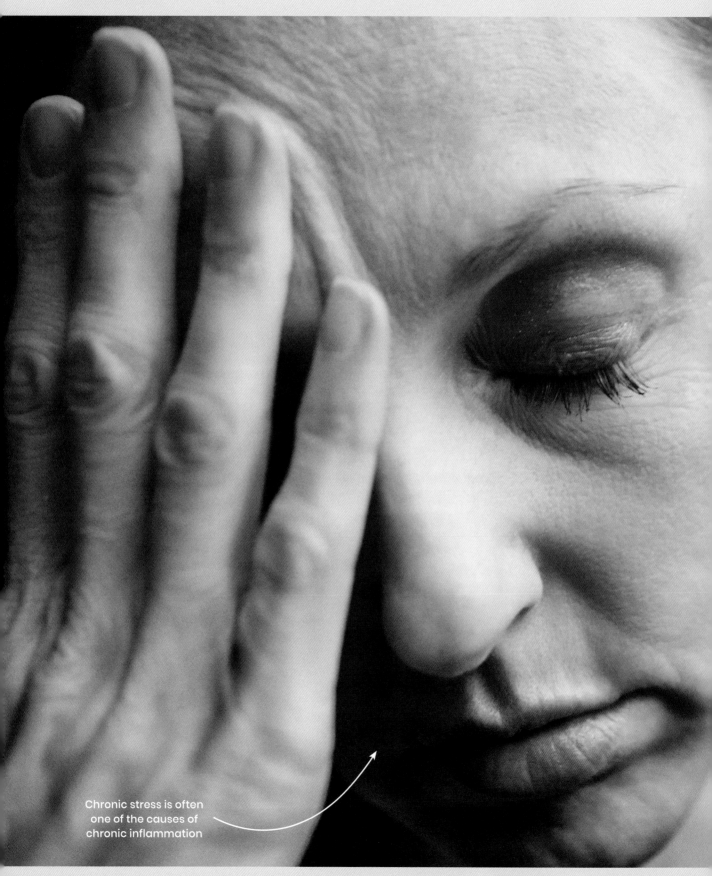

Chronic stress is often one of the causes of chronic inflammation

DIAGNOSING CHRONIC INFLAMMATION

WHEN TO GO TO THE DOCTOR AND WHAT THEY MIGHT DO AND ADVISE

In itself, inflammation is not a problem. In fact, it's one of the ways the body copes with stress. That stress can be external – in the past, spotting a lion put the body into flight or fight mode, now it's more likely to be work related – or internal, in response to disease or injury. Healthy inflammation is what doctors call acute stress: it arises in response to a specific cause, lasts an hour, a few days or a week or two at most, and then decreases. Inflammation becomes unhealthy when it is what doctors call 'chronic'. That means that it lingers on, becoming a constant background to the body's working.

This is also the clue as to when to go to the doctor. If your symptoms have dragged on for weeks or months, often low level but draining, then it is time to make an appointment with your GP.

As inflammation can occur throughout the body, it has many potential symptoms: chronic fatigue, recurring infections, weight gain, weight loss, depression, anxiety, local or general pain, diarrhoea, constipation, rashes and low energy. It really is the ultimate feel-bad-but-not-in-any-specific-way condition.

When you go to the doctor, he or she will try to diagnose you based on your symptoms but, in some cases, it might be necessary to send you for further tests. There is no one specific test for chronic inflammation. Instead, a number of tests check for various markers of inflammation in the body, usually working from a small sample of blood.

Your GP is, in these cases, the first person to see. Because chronic inflammation presents such a wide range of symptoms and because these can all be symptoms of other conditions too, your doctor might have to send you to a specialist, such as a rheumatologist, for further diagnosis.

Should the diagnosis be chronic inflammation, then you are likely to be given a range of treatments. But be sure to be guided by your doctor in this. Your doctor will have your test results, your specific symptoms and your medical history to guide the treatments prescribed; the strategies outlined in this book are much more general and, inevitably, not tailored to any specific reader.

Treatments are likely to include changes in lifestyle, in particular an increase in the amount and types of exercise you do, changes in diet and strategies to improve the quality and quantity of your sleep, as well as various drugs, ranging from over-the-counter NSAIDS (non-steroidal anti-inflammatory drugs), such as ibuprofen and aspirin, to steroids, and DMARDS (disease-modifying anti-rheumatic drugs).

Please remember: this book is a guide but your doctor is the expert. Follow their advice.

Your friendly neighbourhood GP should be your first port of call if you think you're suffering from chronic inflammation

Images Getty, Alamy

31

INFLAMMATORY DISORDERS

What happens when the immune system's responses cause more medical troubles than they cure?

Short-term inflammation is a natural and helpful part of the immune response to threat. When you get a stuffy nose during a cold that is inflammation. This passes quickly and leaves no long-term effects. In inflammatory disorders however the inflammation lingers and causes difficulties for the body which can, in the worst cases, be life changing or even deadly. Inflammatory disorders see the immune system turning against the body and often feature reactions to the body's own cells and chemicals. Even when inflammation does not threaten our physical health it can have a severe impact on our mental health.

1 ASTHMA

Millions of people around the world suffer from asthma, making it one of the most common chronic inflammatory disorders. When a trigger substance enters the lungs of someone with asthma it provokes an immune response which causes the distressing symptoms of an asthma attack. The inflammation that develops causes the airways to swell, the muscles to tighten, and excess mucus to be produced. All of these restrict the amount of air which can be taken into the lungs and makes the asthmatic feel as if they are suffocating. In some cases the inflammation is so severe that breathing becomes impossible and it creates a medical emergency in need of urgent treatment.

Asthma can be treated by avoiding known triggers, like smoke, and through the use of medications. An inhaler may be used every day to lessen the risk of an asthma attack, or when a person feels an attack is starting.

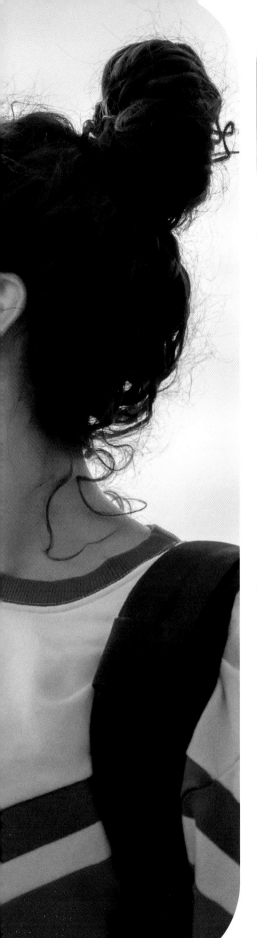

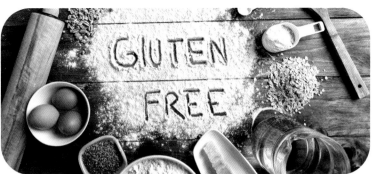

② AUTOIMMUNE DISEASES

Autoimmune disease is an umbrella term for conditions in which the immune system mistakenly targets the cells and systems of the body. Autoimmune responses have been implicated in a vast range of conditions, some of which can be very serious. In multiple sclerosis antibodies attack the sheaths which surround nerve cells and form lesions, or holes, in the brain where normal functions cease. Lupus sees patients' own immune systems targeting multiple tissues and organs throughout the body causing fever, pain, rashes, and tiredness. Coeliac disease is a condition where the immune system reacts to the gluten proteins found in many grains. This triggers the immune system to cause inflammation and also attack cells of the digestive system. Repeated exposure to gluten damages the lining of the small intestine and prevents sufferers taking nutrition from the food they eat. Many autoimmune diseases are incurable but with medication many of those with them can live normal lives.

③ FATTY LIVER DISEASE

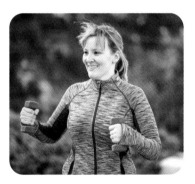

The liver is one of the most important organs in the body and works constantly to process the blood and remove harmful substances. Sometimes too many fat cells form in the liver and this is known as fatty liver disease. Excess alcohol intake can contribute to this but it can happen for no obvious reason. If these fat cells cause inflammation then serious problems can follow. The long-term inflammation creates scar tissue which lacks the vital functions of normal liver tissue. When there is widespread scarring it is known as cirrhosis and can lead to liver failure. If this happens the only available treatment is a liver transplant. For currently unknown reasons fatty livers are more likely to become cancerous.

To reduce your risk of developing fatty liver disease you should reduce or avoid alcohol consumption, reach your target weight, exercise regularly and eat a healthy diet.

4 ALLERGIES

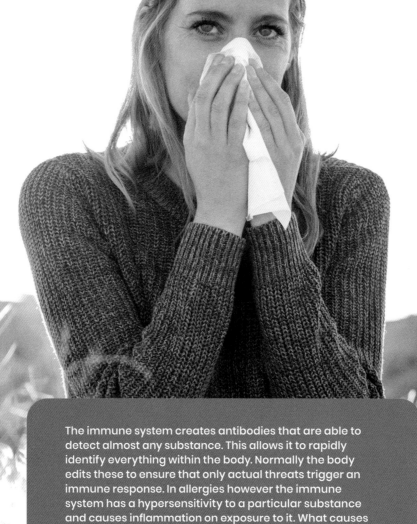

The immune system creates antibodies that are able to detect almost any substance. This allows it to rapidly identify everything within the body. Normally the body edits these to ensure that only actual threats trigger an immune response. In allergies however the immune system has a hypersensitivity to a particular substance and causes inflammation on exposure to it. What causes some people to have allergic reactions is not entirely clear.

Allergies can be as mild as a stuffy nose, sneezing or itchy eyes caused by hayfever. An allergic reaction can, in severe cases, cause anaphylaxis which sees extreme symptoms develop and can be life threatening. Parts of the body can swell with extreme inflammation when triggered. Patients in anaphylaxis can lose the ability to breathe as their lungs swell. A drop in blood pressure can cause them to lose consciousness. Without prompt treatment with medication, such as adrenalin, anaphylaxis can be deadly.

⑤ DIABETES

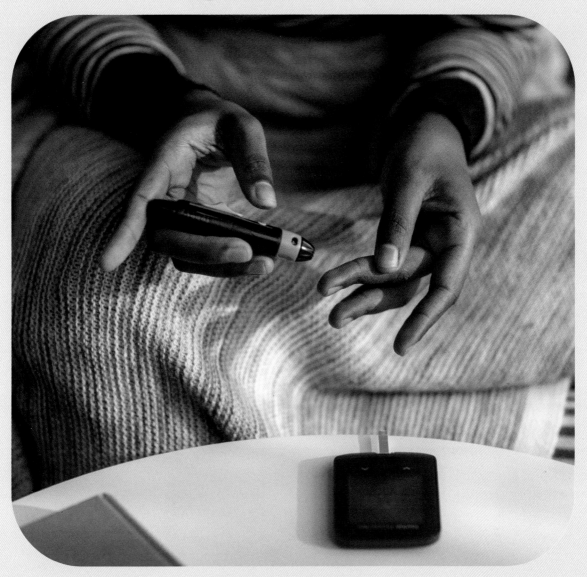

Diabetes is a disease which impairs the ability of the body to regulate levels of glucose in the blood. Normally this is a function of the pancreas and is mediated by the release of the hormone insulin. We need a certain level of glucose in the blood to allow metabolic functions to occur. In diabetes, high levels of glucose cause damage to the small blood vessels and can lead to blindness, numbness, and an inability to heal wounds.

Type 1 diabetes is caused when the insulin-producing cells of the pancreas are lost. Often there is no obvious cause but sometimes it is due to the immune system mistakenly attacking the cells. Without naturally produced insulin the only treatment is regular administration of insulin injections every day.

In type 2 diabetes the body is either unable to produce sufficient insulin or cannot react to the insulin that is produced.

This leads to high levels of blood glucose. People with type 2 diabetes are known to have higher levels of cytokines, the chemical messengers which cause an inflammatory response. It is unknown whether the chronic inflammation is a cause of the diabetes or a result of it. A healthier diet and increased exercise has been proved to both help prevent and treat diabetes, as well as lowering inflammation.

6 ARTHRITIS

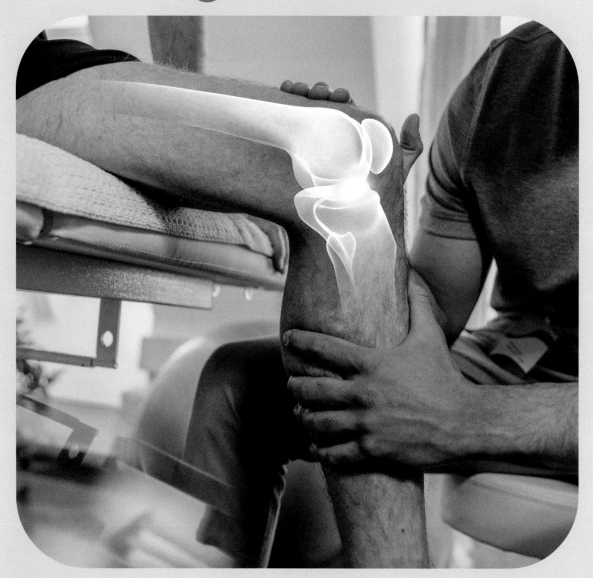

Arthritis is the name for a variety of conditions that see people suffering pain and swelling in the joints of their bodies. Normally these joints are protected and cushioned by pads of cartilage which help the bones to move smoothly next to each other. In arthritis the cartilage becomes ineffective and the bones begin to rub against each other. When this occurs there can be a great deal of pain and the flesh around the joint can swell massively. Loss of ability to use the joint normally is common.

Some types of arthritis, like osteoarthritis, have relatively low levels of inflammation but some, like rheumatoid arthritis, are directly caused by inflammation. In inflammatory arthritis the immune system targets the thin membranes around the joints and causes swelling that leads to stiffness and pain. The irritation caused by the inflammation leads to the disintegration of the cartilage in the joints and worsens the symptoms. As the hands are often the site of rheumatoid arthritis, an attack of it can leave patients unable to perform their normal daily tasks.

Treatments can help to manage the disease by reducing the pain and swelling, but there is currently no cure.

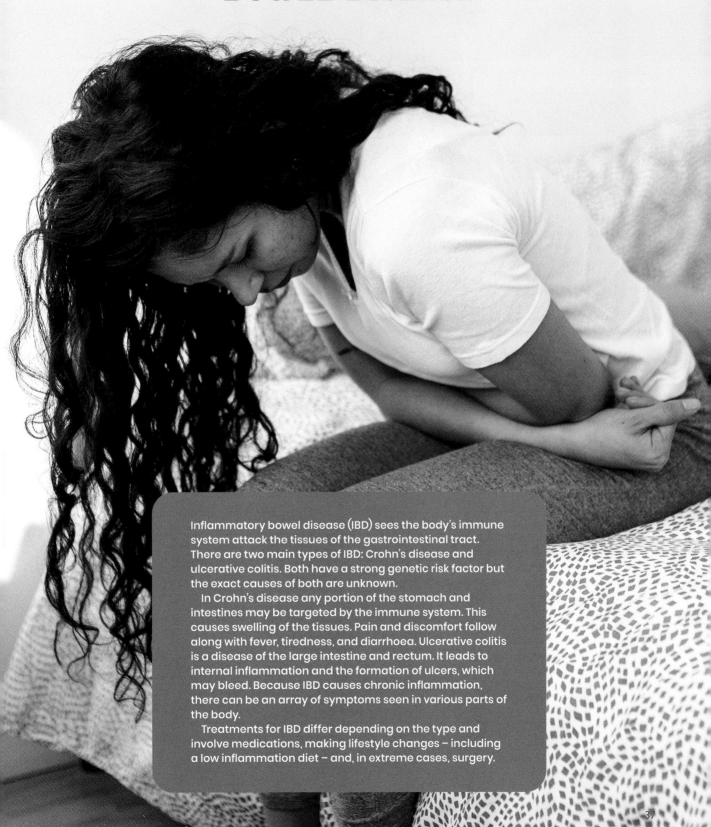

7 INFLAMMATORY BOWEL DISEASE

Inflammatory bowel disease (IBD) sees the body's immune system attack the tissues of the gastrointestinal tract. There are two main types of IBD: Crohn's disease and ulcerative colitis. Both have a strong genetic risk factor but the exact causes of both are unknown.

In Crohn's disease any portion of the stomach and intestines may be targeted by the immune system. This causes swelling of the tissues. Pain and discomfort follow along with fever, tiredness, and diarrhoea. Ulcerative colitis is a disease of the large intestine and rectum. It leads to internal inflammation and the formation of ulcers, which may bleed. Because IBD causes chronic inflammation, there can be an array of symptoms seen in various parts of the body.

Treatments for IBD differ depending on the type and involve medications, making lifestyle changes – including a low inflammation diet – and, in extreme cases, surgery.

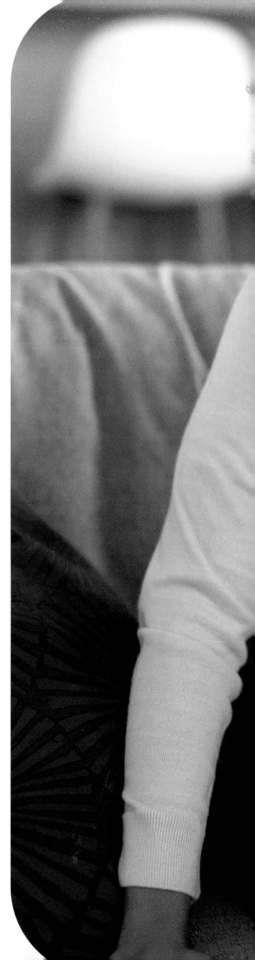

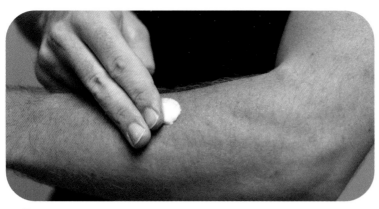

8 DERMATITIS

Dermatitis is a medical term that refers to any inflammation of the skin. It can have many causes and a variety of symptoms but all involve an inflammatory response that often causes discomfort such as irritation, itchiness, redness, flaky patches and soreness. Some types of dermatitis can cause small, itchy blisters to form.

Contact dermatitis is caused by exposure to a specific irritant that triggers the immune system. The substance may cause damage to the cells of the skin, which the immune system responds to as if you have been wounded. It may also be an allergen which directly triggers an immune response.

The best way to avoid dermatitis is to learn which substances trigger it for you and reduce your contact with them as much as possible. Caring for your skin and reducing breaks or cracks may help as well.

9 PERIODONTITIS

Periodontitis, also known as periodontal disease, is a distressing condition where bacterial presence near the teeth causes inflammation of the gums. The immune response to the bacteria leads to swelling, pain, and redness in the earliest stages.

Over time the chronic inflammation can make the gums recede from the teeth. Upon brushing the teeth, the gums can become further irritated, tender and begin to bleed. The bone around the teeth can soften as well, which can cause the teeth to become sensitive, or even loose and eventually fall out. Because of the bacteria, people with periodontal disease may suffer from persistent bad breath.

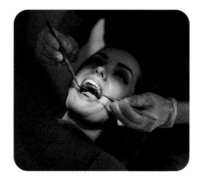

The best way to avoid periodontitis is to ensure you brush thoroughly and maintain optimum oral health. Regular trips to the dentist will help you identify if the problem is beginning. Smoking has been proved to be associated with periodontitis so stopping smoking may reduce your risk.

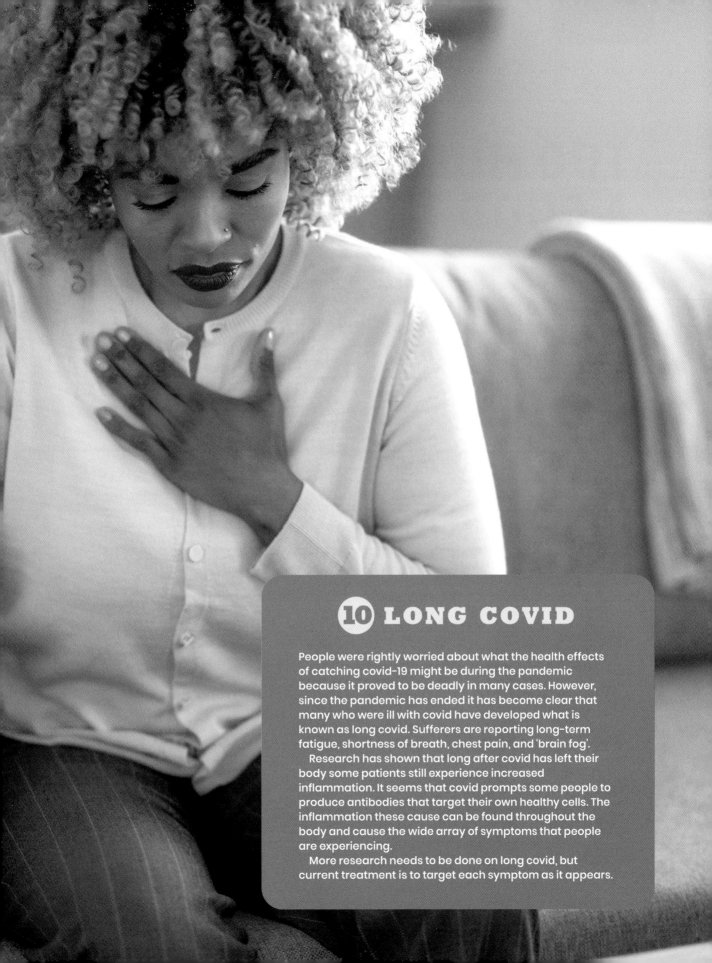

⑩ LONG COVID

People were rightly worried about what the health effects of catching covid-19 might be during the pandemic because it proved to be deadly in many cases. However, since the pandemic has ended it has become clear that many who were ill with covid have developed what is known as long covid. Sufferers are reporting long-term fatigue, shortness of breath, chest pain, and 'brain fog'.

Research has shown that long after covid has left their body some patients still experience increased inflammation. It seems that covid prompts some people to produce antibodies that target their own healthy cells. The inflammation these cause can be found throughout the body and cause the wide array of symptoms that people are experiencing.

More research needs to be done on long covid, but current treatment is to target each symptom as it appears.

TOO MUCH OF A GOOD THING

Inflammation is a natural response to disease and injury but sometimes it lingers long after it should... and then it becomes dangerous

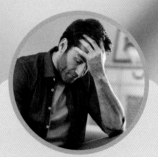

Trap your finger in a door and, after screaming and shouting for a while, you will see the finger starting to swell. The swelling is the visible indicator of the body's response to harm. It's a dangerous world out there – the body can suffer damage from physical injuries, bacteria, viruses, poisons and toxins. As such, the body has developed many strategies for dealing with injuries. The first to respond are the body's emergency services, inflammatory cells and cytokines, which produce more inflammatory cells.

The aim is to keep the damage local, trapping bacteria or stopping the trauma from injury spreading further. Within the inflamed area, the body sets about repairing damaged tissue and hunting for invading pathogens, targetting them with white blood cells.

This is a perfectly normal response and it produces the acute inflammation associated with injury and disease. In medical terms, acute conditions develop suddenly and go just as quickly. In these cases, inflammation is a welcome thing, as it helps the body to heal.

However, there is another sort of inflammation – chronic inflammation – that is not nearly so helpful. Chronic medical conditions start slowly and last for a long time, so the same is usually true of chronic inflammation. Chronic inflammation occurs when the body keeps on cranking up the inflammatory response even when there is no longer any injury or danger. One example is rheumatoid arthritis, where joint tissues become inflamed through an unwarranted inflammatory response.

Chronic inflammation makes the body think it is under constant attack, so it pumps out white blood cells and other chemicals to deal with the infection. But with no infection to fight, these cells can end up attacking the body itself, causing more inflammation and creating a vicious circle.

Stress is a leading cause of chronic inflammation. Nobody can function when under constant stress but unfortunately the stress of modern life has been linked to a host of physical and psychological conditions. It underlies many of the most common modern pathologies, therefore reducing levels of stress is greatly beneficial to health.

CONDITIONS AND DISEASES LINKED TO CHRONIC INFLAMMATION

Health problems associated with chronic inflammation include:

- Fatty liver disease
- Heart disease
- Type I diabetes
- Type II diabetes
- Cancer
- Rheumatoid arthritis
- Endometriosis
- Inflammatory bowel diseases
- Asthma
- Obesity
- Alzheimer's and Parkinson's disease

Many of these conditions develop from the chronic inflammation that is associated with chronic stress. Looking at ways to reduce stress and inflammation in your life is a key way to improve your health.

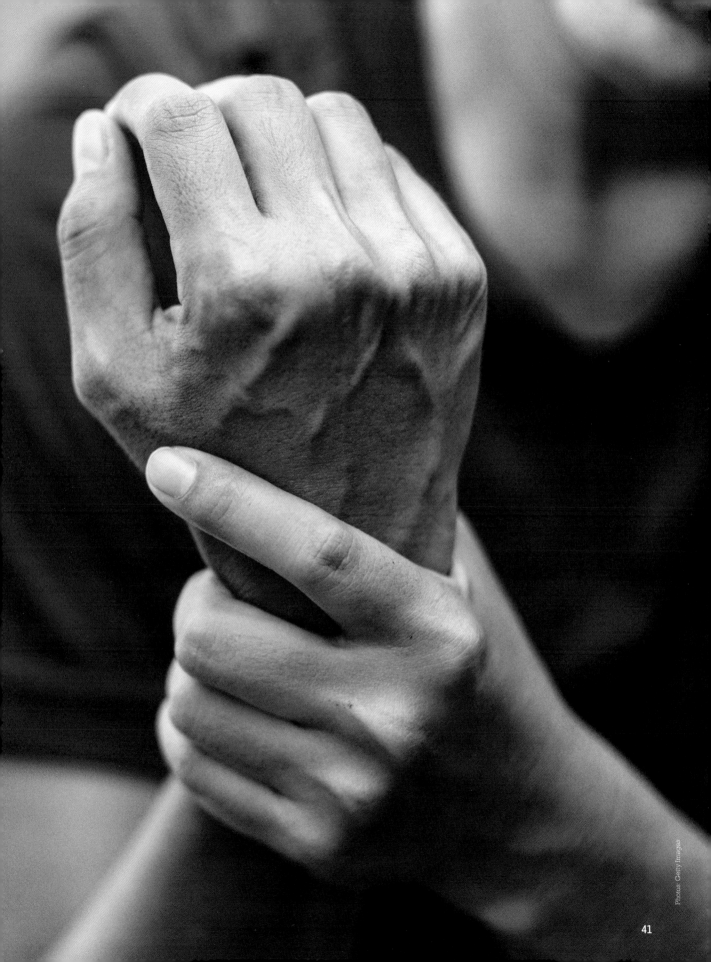

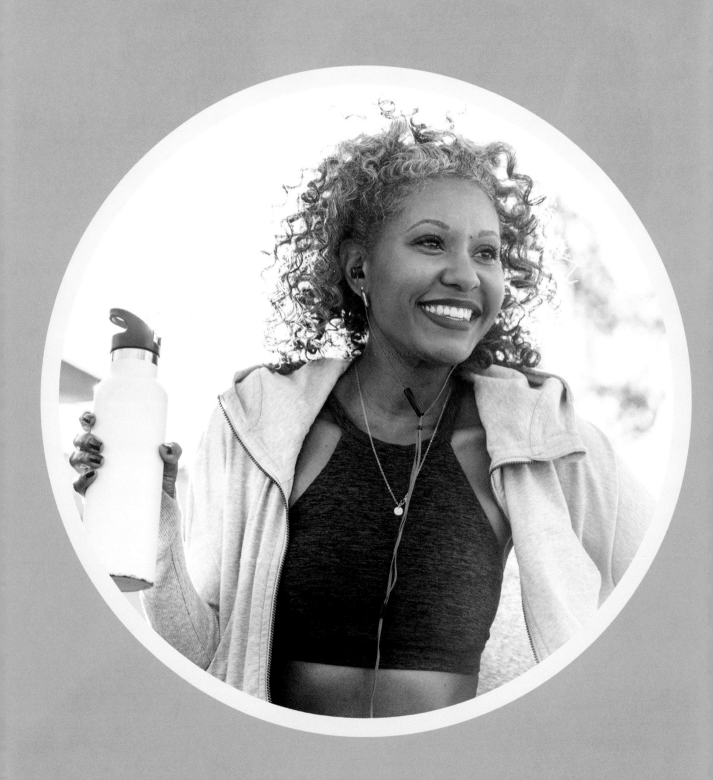

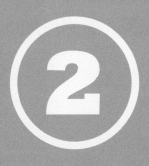

LIFESTYLE

//

*Explore some of the changes you can make
to reduce your risk of chronic inflammation.
Try out a range of exercises, and get tips for
managing stress and improving sleep.*

HEALTHY HABITS

There are lots of things you can do to alleviate inflammation, and most of them will make your life better too

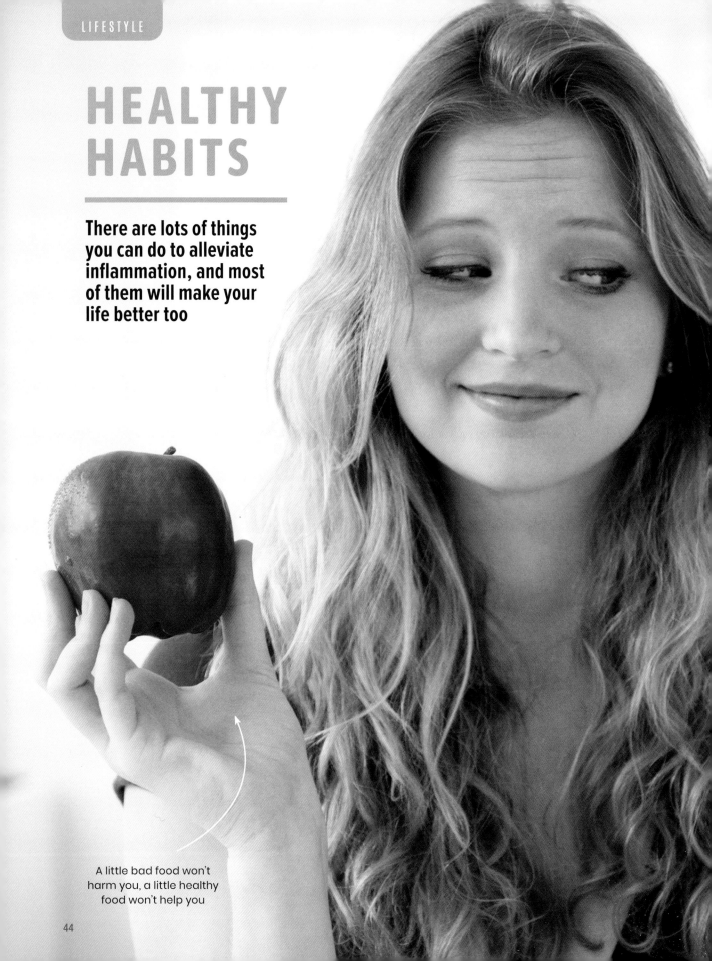

A little bad food won't harm you, a little healthy food won't help you

For people struggling against chronic inflammation, it can sometimes seem as if there is no good news. All too often, a small improvement in one area is accompanied by things getting worse elsewhere.

However, there is one area in which the news is good. There are ways in which we can help the body fight back against chronic inflammation and, what's more, these will also aid our overall health and wellbeing. But in the same way that inflammation tends to creep up slowly, getting worse over weeks, months and years, there are no quick-fix solutions. Nevertheless, by changing what we eat, what we do and how we think, we will reap long-term benefits physically, mentally and even spiritually.

Let's start with what goes into our bodies. There's mounting evidence that some foods contribute to chronic inflammation while other foods act against inflammation. What's even better, the types of food that act against inflammation are often also less fattening – and there's not many people in today's world who couldn't do with losing a pound or two in weight.

To start with, as far as possible, replace processed foods with fresh foods. Think of a typical grocery store, with trays of fresh fruit and vegetables stacked outside and packets and prepared meals inside. Go for the stuff that's outside. Fresh vegetables (frozen vegetables are a reasonable substitute if it's hard to find or store fresh vegetables), fresh fruit and unprocessed meat and fish: these are the basis of a healthy diet. In particular, avoid microwave meals and processed meats. A simple rule of thumb is that food you cook is better for you than food you heat up. Fresh foods come with a whole range of vitamins and minerals that are removed during food processing, as well as lacking the various chemicals that are added to food during processing. What's more, they taste better too! So, that's a win-win right there.

Apart from processed foods, the other huge change from what our ancestors ate is the amount of sugar we consume. Humans, and many other animals, are genetically predisposed towards having sweet teeth because sweet foods are high energy. The difference is that for most of human history, sweet foods were rare: honey, fruit, and that was about it. But with the production of industrial quantities of sugar,

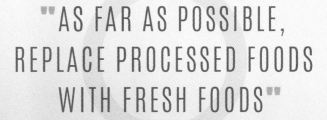

"AS FAR AS POSSIBLE, REPLACE PROCESSED FOODS WITH FRESH FOODS"

we have indulged our fondness for sugar like bears let loose in a honey factory. Today, sugar is added to almost everything. Unfortunately, in these sorts of quantities, sugar becomes inflammatory. So try to reduce your sugar intake. Don't worry. Doing so will make the sugar you do eat taste all the sweeter.

As far as drinking is concerned, take water as the elixir against inflammation. Because many of our modern drinks, from coffee to fizzy drinks and even some fruit juices, are not effective in hydrating the body, a sizeable part of the population remain effectively dehydrated despite drinking cups of coffee and downing cans of cola. A dehydrated body is a body under stress – and we all know the part stress plays in inflammation. Drink water, lots of water, to ensure your body is effectively hydrated. Yes, that will mean having to go to the toilet more often but doing so also means that your kidneys are flushing the toxins out of your body faster.

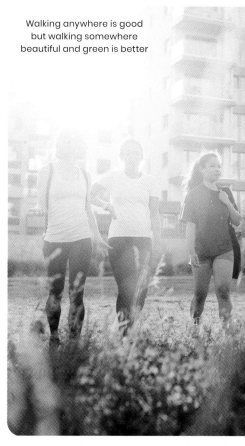

Walking anywhere is good but walking somewhere beautiful and green is better

Having covered what we eat and drink, let's move on to what we do. Or, in the case of sleep, what we don't do. Along with a good diet, sleep is vital. It's only in the last decade or so that scientists have begun to penetrate the mystery of sleep but we have come to understand that having an adequate amount of

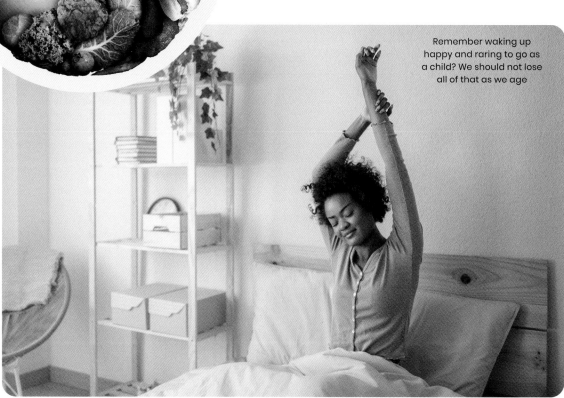

Remember waking up happy and raring to go as a child? We should not lose all of that as we age

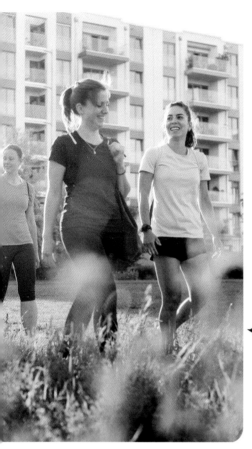

SPICE UP YOUR LIFE

The good news about food is that while we should cut out processed foods, the spices and herbs that make food taste better are, basically, all good for us. Yes, all those Mediterranean herbs and Indian spices produce significant health benefits, from garlic reducing cholesterol to turmeric's pronounced anti-inflammatory properties. Herbs and spices have always been said to be good for health, and research suggests that these claims are true. So spice up your food and spread herbs over your dinner: they will make the food taste better and do you good as well. Another win-win!

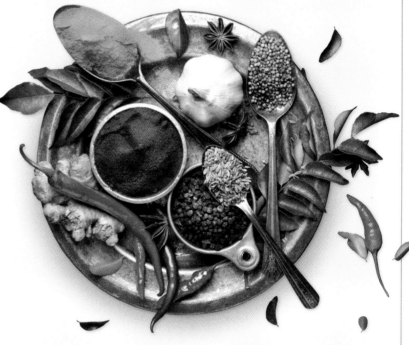

quality shut-eye is essential for well-being. We really do need eight hours of sleep a night. It is true, there are some people who can function productively with less but, in doing so, they gamble on their future health.

To facilitate a good night's sleep, switch off all electronic devices at least an hour before bedtime and develop a regular sleep routine, going to bed at roughly the same time each night. Avoid stimulating drinks and food for at least a couple of hours before retiring and try to ensure your bedroom is cool and dark. Doing so will help to ensure a good night's sleep, when the body can go about fixing the strains and stresses of the day.

Making sure you have a good night's sleep will not only help to make the day brighter and more productive, it will help you live longer. Several studies have now shown that lack of sleep is linked to shorter lifespans. So not only does sleep make the day better, it helps you live longer too. If that's not a win win, nothing is!

However, many people today have problems with getting and staying asleep. Another way of helping to achieve those elusive eight hours is by exercising earlier in the day (not just before bed as that will make it harder to get to sleep). But that's only one of the benefits of exercise.

Our bodies were made to move. For the vast majority of human existence we were nomads, moving from a hunting site to a forest where the apples were ripe. We are made to walk. Modern, sedentary life is almost designed to be unhealthy, from the postural difficulties of spending too long sitting down to the biochemical changes that produce obesity, heart disease and osteoporosis. Therefore, it should come as no surprise that the life of a couch potato is prone to chronic inflammation. The solution, exercise, is obvious, the practice in today's world much less so.

Images Getty, Alamy

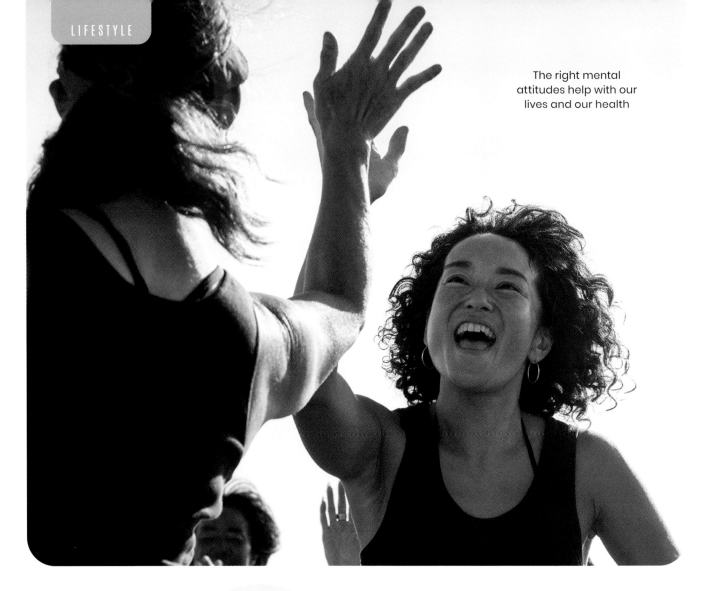

The right mental attitudes help with our lives and our health

"IMPROVING BALANCE HAS THE SIDE EFFECT OF INCREASING CONFIDENCE IN MOVEMENT"

However, the key is to remember that we were made for movement. We might be tied to a desk but that does not stop us standing up every half hour, stretching and moving around a little. If possible, invest in a standing desk. And when going to and from the office, maximise movement: take the stairs rather than the lift, discover the area with a lunchtime walk, go and see a colleague rather than pinging them an email. Of all forms of exercise, walking is the most easily and thoroughly beneficial (although swimming runs it close). However, you don't have to towel yourself dry after going for a walk.

Any form of exercise is beneficial, although be careful not to overdo things at the start. As we age, it's also worth adding forms of exercise that improve balance to your routine, such as yoga or tai chi. Balance is probably the most undervalued form of fitness but its value increases greatly as we get older, when falls become potentially more dangerous. Improving balance has the side effect of increasing confidence in movement, allowing us to keep mobile – age-related obesity is often associated with increased fear of falling as a result of a lessening sense of balance.

Doing what we were designed to do – move – not only makes our bodies work better, it makes

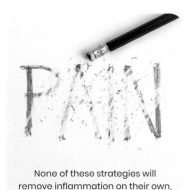

None of these strategies will remove inflammation on their own, but carry them out together and they will slowly reduce the pain

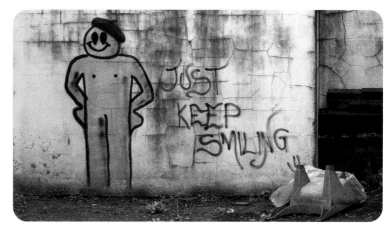

us feel better too. Which brings us to what we think and how that affects us.

The body and the mind are not separate. We all know how a lingering illness can drag our mood down. But the same works in the opposite direction: a happy and positive mind will experience the same set of physical difficulties differently to someone who is unhappy and depressed. This principle is embedded in every drug trial: placebos produce a positive medical effect even though they contain no drug. Belief has a proven medical benefit.

So do optimism and happiness. Numerous studies have shown that people who are optimistic and happy have better health outcomes than people who are pessimistic and depressed – they even live longer!

While for most people it's not possible to just flip the happiness switch, cultivating attitudes of mind that emphasise gratitude and hope, engagement, meaning, positive social relationships and achievement for its own sake will gradually produce a shift in mental attitude. These are perhaps the ultimate win win, as they enable us to deal with life's transitions in a better way. We cannot change the world, but we can change how we experience the world. Do that well, and everything else will follow.

A LIFE IN BALANCE

Chronic inflammation is one sign of a body, and a life, out of balance. Restoring that balance is a crucial part of the strategy to reverse the effects of chronic inflammation. To do so, we need to look at ourselves, and our lives, on the whole. There is no magic inflammation pill that will put everything right. Instead, we need to put in place different strategies to restore balance to our lives, from eating better and sleeping longer through to exercising more and cultivating the right mental attitudes. But the good news is that doing this will not only reduce inflammation, it will make everything else in our lives better too.

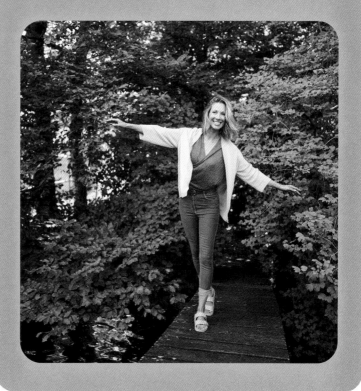

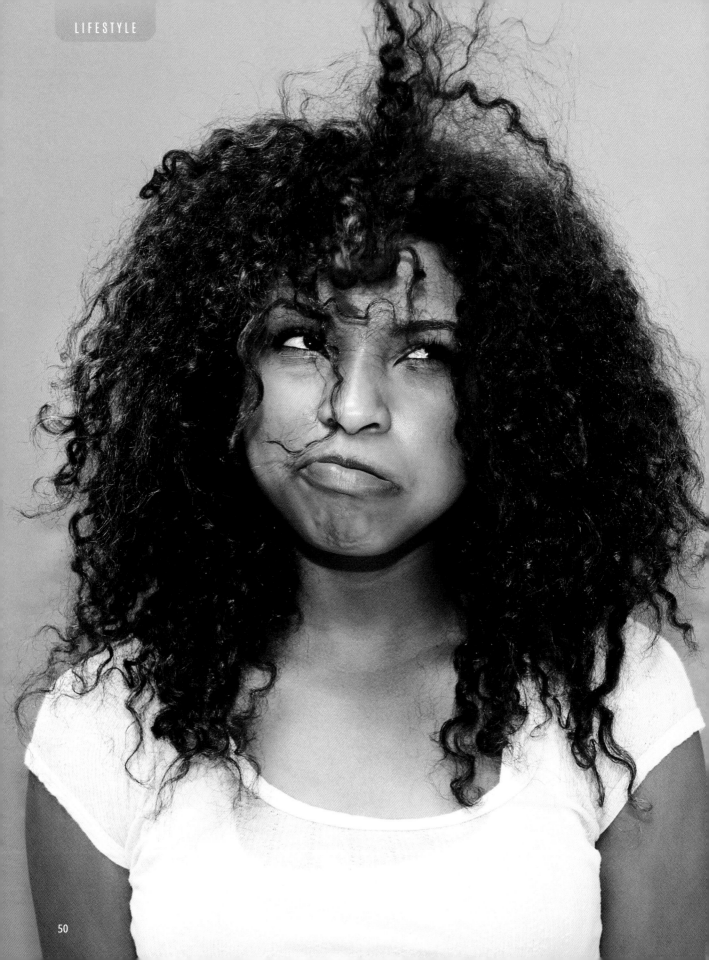

STOP STRESSING

Why the body needs stress and what to do when it gets too much of it

A hundred thousand years ago, when our ancestors were walking the plains of Africa, the sight of the savannah grass rippling when there was no wind sent a spike of adrenaline through their bodies: a lion might be on the hunt.

The acute stress triggered by spotting a stalking lion triggers the body's fight or flight response. Stress hormones are released, of which the main one is cortisol. Cortisol produces energy and regulates the immune system. All well and good should we realise that the waving grass was just a wandering breeze, as that allows the cortisol production to tail off and the body return to normal. Not so good if the body doesn't get the all-clear signal.

Which is where chronic stress comes in. The body reacts in the same way to a stalking lion and a bullying boss. But where the lion either attacks or doesn't, we are all too often stuck with the bullying boss. Stress hormones remain elevated. The rest functions of the body are suppressed because we are living in flight-or-fight mode all the time.

We need to give our body downtime. Here are some ways to help it get there.

Getting to sleep

////////////////////

Sleep is good in general but it's particularly good for stress and inflammation. Unfortunately, chronic stress makes getting a good night, or week's, sleep much more difficult. As such, it's worth knowing about some other ways to grab those zzzs beyond the usual advice about a regular bedtime routine and avoiding coffee.

And you know what? There's an app for this. In fact, there are rather a lot of apps out there. Search for sleep apps and you'll find a whole range of which some of the best are Calm, Headspace

and Sleep Easy. These will guide you through meditation and calming techniques designed to help you sleep better. They also have the virtue of doing most of the work for you, so you just have to do what the calm voice says. (Sleep apps are the only exception to the rule that it's best to switch off your phone at least an hour before bedtime.)

Pay attention

////////////////////

The racing mind that accompanies chronic stress can sometimes be slowed and settled by using various grounding

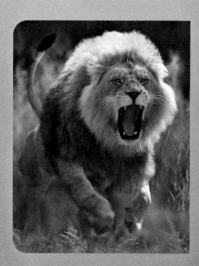

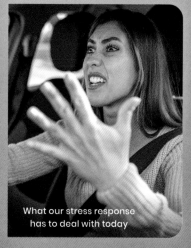

What our stress response has to deal with today

Images Getty, Alamy

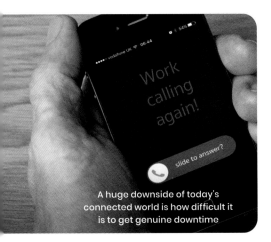

A huge downside of today's connected world is how difficult it is to get genuine downtime

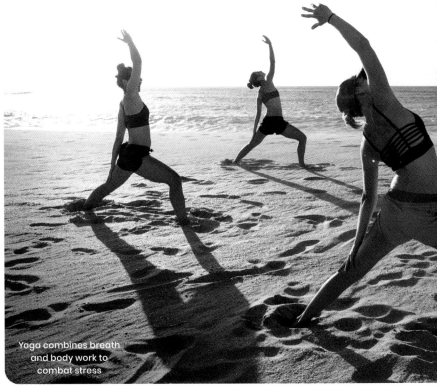

Yoga combines breath and body work to combat stress

techniques. These are all designed to draw the attention away from what is causing stress – whether it's worrying about exams, unpaid bills or reliving ghastly memories – and back into the present moment where, in most cases, we are not immediately threatened.

The 5-4-3-2-1 technique begins with breathing in to a slow count of four and then out to a slow count of four. Maintain this breathing rhythm throughout the exercise.

On the next exhale, say aloud the names of five things you can see from wherever you are. During the next breath, say the names of four things you can hear. For the following breath, it's three things you can feel. Then two things you can smell, and finally one thing you can taste. The point of the exercise is to enter fully into each sense during each breath, concentrating on your immediate surroundings and sensations as a counterweight to the racing of a stressed mind.

The 3-3-3 rule is a similar technique, although this time you first name three things you can see directly, while examining them with complete attention, then listen to three things intently, and finally move three parts of the body, concentrating all your attention on what you are doing.

It's all in the breath

There are many meditation styles that people advocate for reducing stress, but simple breath control is a good place to start. People in a state of chronic stress tend to have faster breathing patterns – after all, they're in a constant state of flight/fight – controlling this is a simple way to switch the body out of this state.

You will see many magazine articles advocating a breath pattern of a long count of four on the inbreath and a count of eight on the outbreath. This does indeed work well in shifting the body to its rest/digest state. However, it's not always effective for people who are highly stressed. In such a state, trying to shift straight away into a state of relaxation may be too big a step. So, if you're feeling particularly stressed, it might be better to begin with an even breathing

rhythm, in for a long count of four and out for a long count of four. This gives the body the chance to pull back from its state of extreme anxiety. When stress has died down somewhat, then it's often a good idea to change to four/eight breathing to nudge the body into its rest/digest state. But often, the first step is simply calming down.

It's all in the mind

You can barely open a magazine today without finding an article about mindfulness. Indeed, it's easy to think that it's the only form of meditation. This is not the case though. There are many different forms and techniques originating from a whole range of the world's spiritual practices as well as coming directly from recent research. So there should be something to suit everyone.

Apart from mindfulness meditation, which basically asks

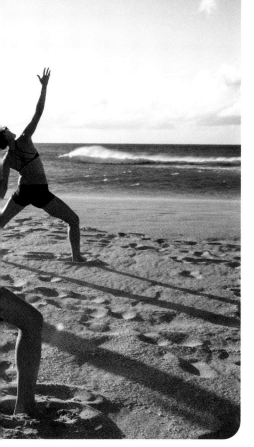

practitioners to pay attention to the passing moment without holding on to it, there are practices that focus on breath, on movement, images and visualisation. All of these techniques have one thing in common: breath control. The conscious control of breathing required in meditation has a direct effect the nervous system by inducing it into a more relaxed state, in turn reducing both stress and inflammation.

Perhaps the easiest form of meditation is guided meditation as, in this case, there's a teacher or narrator to bring your attention back to the meditation when it, inevitably, wanders.

After that, simple breath meditation is probably the next easiest.

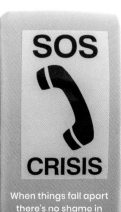

When things fall apart there's no shame in seeking help

Concentrate on your breath, breathing in and breathing out. When attention wanders – and it will – bring it back to your breath. All you will have missed is a few breaths.

These are two excellent starting points for beginners in meditation. But no form of meditation is difficult in principle, although doing them well can be more difficult in practice. Try and see what works best for you.

When it gets overwhelming

It's all very well talking about ways of coping with stress but there are times in life – such as the death of a loved one or losing one's job suddenly – when a few minutes slow breathing is really not going to cut it. In a crisis, even people who have practised all the above techniques for years, can find themselves pushed to breaking point.

At such times there is no shame in seeking help. There are many organisations who can help in a crisis, depending on what the nature of the emergency is. If you are in the depths of a mental health crisis, the NHS has urgent mental health helplines, open 24 hours a day, where you can speak to a mental health professional who will help decide on the best course of action. In the UK, go to **www.nhs.uk** where you will be

asked your location and then given the phone number for your appropriate helpline.

Along with the NHS, there are the Samaritans on 116 123. Alternatively, text SHOUT to 85258 for the Shout Crisis Text Line or, if you are under 19, call Childline on 0800 1111. The mental health charity, Mind, has a complete list of crisis helplines: **www.mind.org.uk**.

Crises can come in many different forms. If it's financial, then you can get help and advice from the Citizen's Advice Bureau as well as helplines such as Money Helper (0800 011 3797), National Debtline (0808 808 4000) and StepChange Debt Charity (0800 138 1111).

Bereavement can seem overwhelming. If you need help, try calling the National Bereavement Service on 0800 0246 121 or the Good Grief Trust at **www.thegoodgrieftrust.org**. If you're outside the UK, search online for local services and helplines in your area.

Stopping stress

The simple truth is that life is stressful and nobody escapes entirely unscathed! But while we can't escape the troubles and tragedies of life, we can, perhaps, modify how we experience them. These are all suggestions that might help but you are your own best guide as to what is most effective for you.

LEARNING TO RELAX

Discovering a new way of self-soothing – be it with an activity or natural medication – can swiftly reduce stress levels. So what will suit you best?

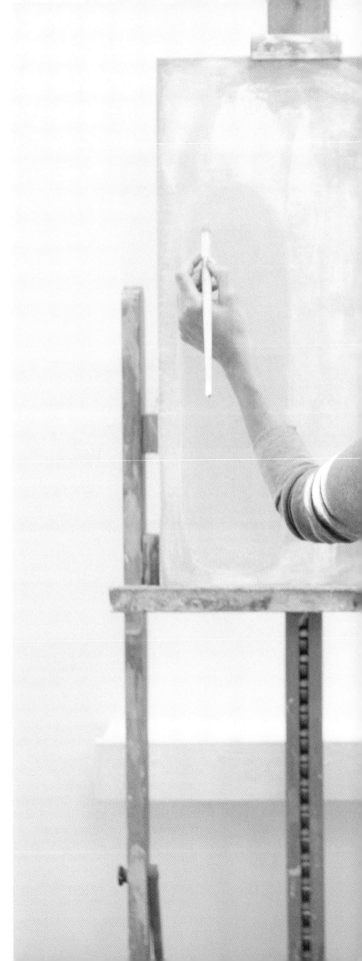

R elaxation is an essential addition to our wellbeing toolkit, but it's not always easy to accomplish, especially in challenging circumstances. But learning to do it right could help reduce stress and inflammation in our bodies.

'Relaxation is vital to our health and wellbeing, as well as our immune function,' says natural health and wellness expert Dr Tim Bond. 'Researchers at Harvard Medical School discovered that in people practising relaxation methods, such as yoga and meditation, far more "disease-fighting genes" were active, compared to those who didn't practise. In particular, they found genes were switched on that help to protect from disorders such as pain, infertility, high blood pressure and even rheumatoid arthritis.'

And that's not all. The art of relaxation also drives higher levels of feel-good chemicals, such as serotonin and growth hormones, which repair cells and tissue. 'In essence, relaxation has virtually the opposite effect to stress, lowering heart rate, boosting immunity and enabling the body to thrive,' says Dr Bond. 'An example is when women menstruate, they often find taking a long bath or doing some gentle relaxation exercises helps their general wellbeing.'

Sounds great, but our hectic lives often prevent us from finding – and utilising – what's best for us. In order to move away from the sympathetic (fight or flight) response and activate the parasympathetic (rest and digest) response, we must trust our instincts and choose what produces

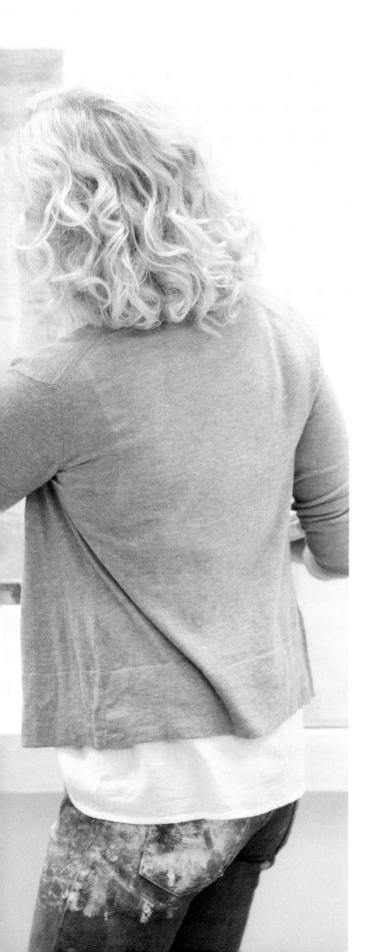

the most satisfaction. 'It's about finding out what's right for you,' says Dr Megan Jones Bell, chief science officer at Headspace (headspace.com). 'Breathing can be a powerful way to help us reset and activate our natural relaxation response, so one of the easiest and most accessible ways for anyone to relax, in any setting, environment or activity, is to focus on the breath.'

As well as spending time in nature, playing with animals, getting a massage, and praying or meditating, here are some quick and effective ways to put you back on the path to wellness.

The art of... creating

Creating can be anything, from taking an art class or colouring in, to crafts or jigsaw puzzles. These forms of active mediation allow us to settle our overworked brains and focus on the here and now. 'Art has the power to heal, increase wellbeing and reduce anxiety. Researchers liken creating art to exercise for the brain, and studies consistently show that creating art helps individuals cope with stressful and difficult situations,' says Scott Phillips, co-founder of Rise Art (riseart.com).

Even doodling is beneficial. Writing in Psychology Today (psychologytoday.com), Cathy Malchiodi, PhD, says: 'The wonderful thing about doodling is that it is a whole-brain activity – self-soothing, satisfying, exploratory and mindful.'

The art of... yogic breathing

Brighton-based yoga practitioner Danny Griffiths (yoga-fit.co.uk) recommends alternate nostril breathing, called nadi shodhana pranayama. It activates the parasympathetic response, strengthening the immune system and providing quick relief from stress.

She says, 'I do this before classes, as I find it really relaxing and calming. It's meant to balance the "ida" and "pingala" nadis (channels) or the yin and the yang.' Explaining how to do it, she says, 'Sit up straight in a cross-legged position with your left hand resting on your thigh, exhale completely then use your right thumb to close your right nostril. Inhale for four to five seconds through your left nostril then close this nostril with

THE ART OF... SOUND THERAPY

Sound therapy has been used for centuries to help people enter a more relaxed, meditative state, and promote wellbeing and healing. Now, thanks to modern technology, there's a new-ish kid on the block – binaural beats. Through headphones, listeners receive a different sound frequency to each ear, which the brain interprets as a particular rhythmic frequency. These sounds create specific neural responses that induce one of five brainwave states that can aid sleep and ease pain (delta brainwaves), help you relax or meditate (theta), reduce stress (alpha), improve concentration and focus (beta), and enhance memory (gamma). neuroscientists, it's so effective that it's strongly recommended that you don't drive while listening!

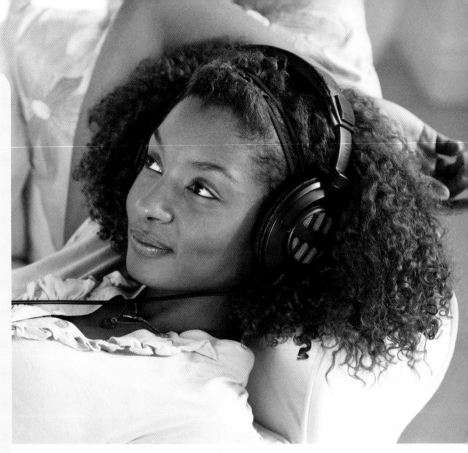

your ring finger and exhale for four to five seconds through your right nostril. Inhale through the right nostril then close it with your thumb and breathe out through the left nostril. Repeat for three to five minutes. Finish on the left nostril.'

While this type of breathing can be done at any time, it's worth combining with yoga. 'Yoga is more of a work-in than work-out,' says Danny. 'Classes are meditative as we move from posture to posture, and for some students it's the only time they can switch off. After concentrating on how the body feels in the moment, there's no denying the state of relaxation at the end of practice.'

The art of... organising

//////////////

If your mother ever said "tidy house, tidy mind", she wasn't just trying to persuade you to clean your room – the chances are she recognised the positive effects of an ordered environment. And, with many of us taking staycations, it's more important than ever to create a Zen home.

Research has shown that working up a sweat while cleaning improves mental health and boosts mood, while Japanese organising consultant Marie Kondo waxes lyrical about "a comfortable environment, a space that feels good to be in, a place where you can relax" in her bestseller *The Life-Changing Magic of Tidying Up* (Vermilion).

The art of... ASMR

//////////////////////////

For those who enjoy Autonomous Sensory Meridian Response (ASMR), the experience can be nothing short of profound. ASMR enthusiasts love the de-stressing effects of listening to sounds, such as whispering, eating, a cat purring or rainfall, or by watching kinetic sand or soap being sliced.

The theory behind these stimuli is the release of feel-good chemicals – endorphins, dopamine, oxytocin and serotonin – into our bodies, which decrease stress and aid relaxation. 'ASMR is consistently helpful at bringing comfort, peace and calmness to busy brains when an overactive mind is preventing a desired feeling of calmness. While it can't cure or prevent any form of illness, it may help reduce feelings of stress or sleeplessness,' says Dr Craig Richard, founder of ASMR University (**asmruniversity. com**).

The art of... natural self-medicating with cannabidiol

If you self-medicate with alcohol or drugs, try a natural approach instead – it's better for your body and mental state. 'Quality, tested CBD [cannabidiol] oil like DragonflyCBD (dragonflycbd. com) has been found to bust anxiety and stress, and help users, along with other self-care tips, to get to that deep relaxation state,' explains Dr Bond. 'Evidence from studies has shown that CBD has anti-anxiety effects, may regulate learned fear, and appears to reduce the cardiovascular response to models of stress and reduce resting blood pressure,' he adds.

The art of... salt bathing

Salt baths have long been regarded as an elixir to combat stress and encourage relaxation, and the secret lies in magnesium. 'Individuals who suffer with mental-health illnesses have been found to have lower platelet serotonin levels,' explains Karen Davis, Westlab chief pharmacist (westlabsalts.co.uk). 'There are different ways to increase serotonin, including magnesium intake,' she adds. 'This is best absorbed through the skin.'

That's why a soak in a bath filled with salts rich in magnesium, such

as Dead Sea, Epsom or Himalayan salts, is advised. 'This will not only help to calm and de-stress the mind and body, but also improve mood,' Karen explains.

The art of... everyday mindfulness

Contrary to popular belief, mindfulness isn't about sitting quietly and meditating, which can take time and practice. 'We can introduce relaxation into our daily life by simply trying to be more mindful in our everyday tasks,' explains Dr Jones Bell. 'This could be as simple as mindful hand-washing, making a cup of tea or taking moments to pause and check in with yourself. Rather than getting lost in the frustration of a task, acknowledge it, accept it, sit with it, focus on your breathing and bring your attention back to how you're feeling and why. This will help you be intentional in every interaction and can bring about a more relaxed state of being,' she says.

The art of... neo-Luddism

Neo-Luddites reject modern technology, and so can you. 'Give it a go, even for an hour, and see what difference it makes,' says burnout coach Rosie Millen (**missnutritionist.com**). 'We live in a comparative age, which is not healthy. From the moment we wake up to the moment we go to bed we are reminded of what everyone is doing and achieving in every 24-hour window. This emphasises the need to switch off to get in touch with real life.'

RELAX, IT'S AS EASY AS BREATHING

You breathe 22,000 times a day, and by doing it mindfully, you can free yourself from stress

Y our breath is the greatest asset you have. Of course, its primary function is to keep us alive by bringing oxygen into the body. But it is also naturally meditative. It reflects your most powerful emotions and if you learn to understand it, can either soothe or harness them. There is an art to breathing correctly, and it's one that many of us have forgotten.

How breathing works

Breathing relies on the big, powerful muscles of the diaphragm, the abdomen and the intercostal muscles that lie between the ribs. It is helped along by the smaller secondary muscles of the neck, shoulders and upper ribs.

When you are upset, anxious or stressed, the abdomen tenses and prevents the big primary muscles from working. Instead, they begin tugging against each other, leaving the secondary muscles to do all the work. But the secondary muscles are only designed to shoulder 20 per cent of the burden, so they become stressed. If this continues, it can lead to chronic tension in the shoulders and neck, headaches and fatigue, and increasingly shallower breathing. It's a vicious cycle that lies behind much of our anxiety, stress and unhappiness. But there is an equally powerful virtuous cycle that you can cultivate by learning the art of breathing.It's at the heart of mindfulness and as old as meditation itself. You can learn the basics in just a few minutes, although mastering it takes a little longer.

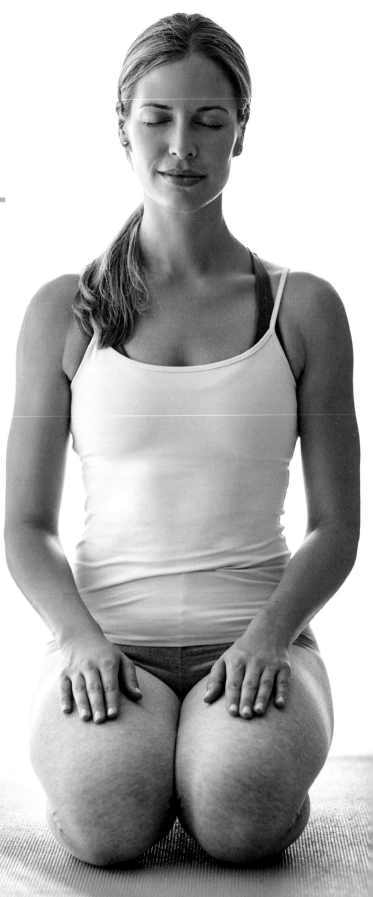

Understanding mindfulness and your mind

//////////////////////////

Mindfulness is simply full, conscious awareness of whatever thoughts, feelings and emotions are flowing through your mind, body and breath without judging or criticising them in any way. It is being fully aware of whatever is happening in the present moment.

The aim of mindfulness is not to clear the mind of thoughts. It is to understand how your mind works. It teaches you to observe how your thoughts and feelings rise and fall like waves. And in the calm spaces lie moments of piercing insight.

You come to learn that happiness is fleeting, while unhappiness lingers. Psychologists call it the negativity bias. It skews perception and makes the world seem far harsher than it actually is.

The negativity bias ensures that it takes five positive experiences to balance a single negative one. It's no more difficult than tuning into the breath while paying attention to the little pleasures of daily life. It means noticing the sights, sounds, smells and textures that surround you, and soaking up the tastes and aromas of everything you consume. And while you do so, gently remind yourself that most of life's difficulties are only half as bad as they appear, while the good things are two or three times as intense.

Listen to your body

//////////////////////////////

Through mindfulness, you will come to learn that thoughts, feelings and emotions are created by the body as much as the brain.

It's called embodied cognition. A fleeting moment of stress, for example, creates tension in the body. The brain senses this and interprets it as stress. The body tenses a little more, breathing becomes a little shallower, the brain feels more stressed. It's a downward spiral.

Mindful breathing will teach you that your most powerful states of mind are reflected in the body as physical sensations. Anxiety might appear as nausea. Stress as a headache. Depression might trigger physical pain – a broken heart, perhaps. Be aware of these sensations – each one is a message.

If you consciously listen to these messages by actively feeling them in your body, you'll realise that they rise and fall like your breath. And before long they'll begin to melt away, leaving behind a calmer, happier and more insightful mind.

Meditate under the stars

///////////////

You'll probably spend 36 minutes worrying today (most people do). Perspective dissolves worry. Instead of worrying, why not go outside and breathe? Even better, gaze at the stars.

Take off your shoes and socks. Feel the ground beneath your feet. Look upwards. Breathe. See the stars streaming off into infinity in every direction.

Focus on your breath. Feel the cool night air washing over you. Look at the stars… those twinkles may have taken billions of years to reach you.

Breathe… love the arriving of the light… breathe.

● *The Art of Breathing* by Dr Danny Penman (HQ) is out now. He is also co-author of the 1.5 million-selling book, *Mindfulness*.

TRY THIS LITTLE MINDFUL BREATHING MEDITATION

All you need is a chair, a body, some air, your mind… that's it

● Sit on a straight-backed chair. Place your feet flat on the floor, your spine 2-3cm from the back of the chair.

● Be comfortable, with a relaxed but straight back. Place your hands loosely in your lap. Close your eyes.

● Focus your mind on your breath as it flows in and out. Feel the sensations the air makes. Feel the rise and fall of your chest and stomach.

● Where are the strongest feelings? Nose, mouth, throat, stomach, chest, shoulders? Pay attention and explore the feelings. Don't try to alter them in any way.

● When your mind wanders, bring it back to your breath. Be kind to yourself. Minds wander. It's what they do. Realising that your mind has wandered and bringing it back to your breath is the meditation. It's a little moment of mindfulness.

● After five or ten minutes, gently open your eyes and take in what you can see, hear, feel and smell.

You can download or stream this Breathing Meditation from franticworld.com/aob

SLEEP IT OFF

A good night's sleep is one of the best treatments for chronic inflammation and its associated conditions

It's only very recently that scientists have begun to unlock the mysteries of what happens when we sleep and many questions still remain. But it turns out that Shakespeare was quite right when he has Macbeth proclaim sleep the "balm of hurt minds, great nature's second course, chief nourisher in life's feast". Sleep really is good for you and, the more we learn, the greater the role we see it playing in maintaining the health of our bodies and minds. The irony is that we are learning this in an era when more and more people are finding it difficult to get enough sleep.

people saying, "I'll sleep when I die," not realising that not getting enough sleep makes it more likely that they will die earlier than they would otherwise. Yes, it's true: various studies have found that people who consistently sleep for less than six hours a night are at increased risk of dying before their peers who manage to catch eight hours of shut-eye a night.

Given that many millions of people in Britain and around the world struggle to get to sleep at night, this is clearly a serious issue. Lack of sleep produces short-term effects as well as long term consequences, ranging from fatigue and irritability to an increased likelihood of developing metabolic disorders such as hypertension, diabetes and obesity.

At the mention of the last three, your chronic inflammation alarm might have sounded. You are right: hypertension, diabetes and obesity are strongly correlated with chronic inflammation too. So let us see how lack of sleep is connected to chronic inflammation.

How lack of sleep contributes to chronic inflammation

The exact pathways by which lack of sleep leads to chronic inflammation are the subject of much continuing research. However, some mechanisms are already becoming clear.

Our bodies have natural circadian rhythms that prepare us for a night of sleep and a day of activity. This rhythm is mediated by the production of hormones, including adenosine, melatonin and cortisol.

Adenosine is the day-time hormone, reaching a peak in the evening as we get tired. Melatonin is affected by declining levels of light and acts as the go-to-sleep hormone. Cortisol is our morning wake-up hormone. However, cortisol has a much wider role,

Why it is difficult to get enough sleep today

Although we are slowly learning the importance of sleep for our health, that message has only started to seep through into the wider culture. You'll still hear

"LACK OF SLEEP PRODUCES SHORT-TERM EFFECTS AS WELL AS LONG TERM CONSEQUENCES"

from acting as the emergency response hormone when we are in danger to regulating metabolism, blood pressure and glucose.

In the normal course of events, cortisol levels reduce during daylight hours so that, when evening approaches, we are ready and able to go to sleep. As the night wears into morning, cortisol levels gradually increase, waking us up and reaching a peak in the morning to help us deal with the day ahead.

Melatonin levels reach a peak between 2 and 4am, while cortisol and adenosine are being broken down in the body. However, one effect of not getting enough sleep is that not enough cortisol and adenosine is broken down, leading to us waking up and still feeling tired (too much adenosine) and unrelaxed (too much cortisol still in our system).

How sleep maintains internal bodily hygiene

/////////////////////

The body makes use of the time we are asleep to maintain what we might call its internal hygiene, clearing out and tidying up. One of the key parts of this tidying process is the removal of some of the undesirable by-products of cellular respiration. Oxygen, the molecule that powers respiration, is strongly reactive and the process of respiration itself can produce molecules known as free radicals that are also highly reactive. Having too many free radicals floating around can lead to cellular and DNA damage, possibly triggering cancer formation.

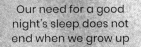

Our need for a good night's sleep does not end when we grow up

To remove these free radicals, the body produces glutathione in the liver, which is a powerful antioxidant. Unfortunately, lack of sleep quite dramatically reduces glutathione production (by 20 to 30 per cent) allowing too many free radicals to continue circulating through the blood stream. Because they are strongly reactive, free radicals end up triggering the body's immune system, contributing to an increase in inflammation and ultimately a state of chronic inflammation.

It's not just free radicals that are flushed out of the system while we are asleep. The brain makes use of this downtime too, increasing the volume of cerebrospinal fluid circulating around the brain and spine, thus removing most of the neurotoxins that accumulate during a hard day's thinking.

Sleep helps you think

There's an old saying: early to bed, early to rise makes Jack healthy, wealthy and wise. We can't vouch for wealth, but health is clearly connected to sufficient sleep. But what about wisdom? That too is connected to sleep, particularly in the learning and retention of new knowledge. Each day we encounter a myriad of new sights, new knowledge and new sensations. The hippocampus region in the brain decides which of these are worthy of retention in our long-term memory.

Many studies, dating from as far back as 1924, have shown that sleep disruption and sleep deficits (when we don't get enough sleep) affect how well we remember new information. There are two main sleep stages, REM and non-REM sleep, and both are necessary for memory formation: REM sleep helps us to remember emotional experiences while non-REM sleep is needed for the accurate retention of words, stories and other information.

Sleep can also be the time when the answers to quandaries that we have been pondering break through into the conscious mind. The chemist August Kekulé had been working on the chemical structure of benzene without success. Then, one night when sleeping, he dreamed of six monkeys dancing and then the six monkeys joined hands and danced in a ring. When he woke up, he knew he had worked out the structure of benzene.

How much sleep do we need?

How much sleep we need depends on age. Infants sleep for between eight and 16 hours a day (new parents will hope their child errs towards the higher end of

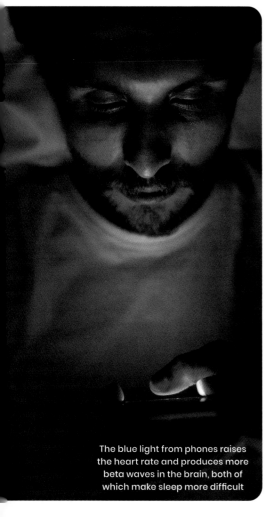

The blue light from phones raises the heart rate and produces more beta waves in the brain, both of which make sleep more difficult

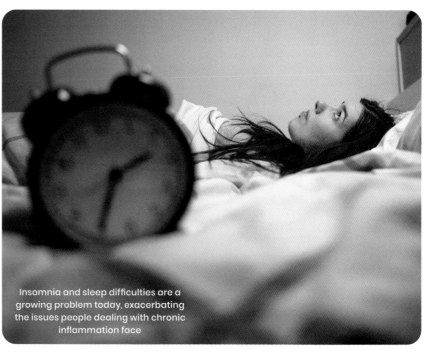

Insomnia and sleep difficulties are a growing problem today, exacerbating the issues people dealing with chronic inflammation face

the scale). For toddlers, the sleep band narrows, to between 11 and 13 hours a day. Younger children (three to five) need 10 to 13 hours, while children between 6 and 12 require nine to 11 hours of sleep. Although they might think otherwise, teenagers still need eight to 10 hours of sleep each night. It's questionable how many actually get all the sleep they need. Adults still require between seven and nine hours of sleep a night. Some people might say they only need four or five hours of sleep, but it's a gamble on their long-term health.

How to get the sleep you need

According to some studies, a third of adults find getting to sleep difficult at least once a week and between six and 10 per cent suffer from clinical insomnia. Sleep problems correlate strongly with the disorders linked to chronic inflammation, including obesity and heart disease. So getting a good night's sleep will help many people on many levels.

If you are suffering chronic sleep problems then it is worth speaking to your doctor. Treatment has moved on a long way from the times when doctors would simply prescribe sleeping pills. However, if your difficulties are more intermittent, it's worth implementing changes to your sleep routine to ensure that there is nothing actively preventing you from getting the sleep you need.

A regular bedtime routine is important. Aim to go to bed at roughly the same time throughout the week. Wildly varying bedtimes throw out the body's natural circadian rhythm. Avoid drinking any stimulants, such as

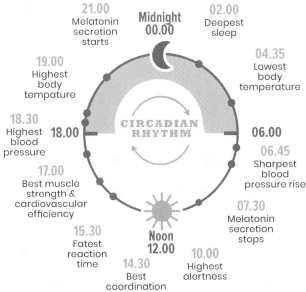

Circadian Rhythm

- **21.00** Melatonin secretion starts
- **Midnight 00.00**
- **02.00** Deepest sleep
- **04.35** Lowest body temperature
- **19.00** Highest body tempature
- **06.00**
- **06.45** Sharpest blood pressure rise
- **18.30** Highest blood pressure
- **18.00**
- **17.00** Best muscle strength & cardiovascular efficiency
- **07.30** Melatonin secretion stops
- **15.30** Fatest reaction time
- **Noon 12.00**
- **10.00** Highest alertness
- **14.30** Best coordination

tea and coffee, for at least two hours before bedtime. Some people are more sensitive to the effects of caffeine and will need to abstain for longer before bedtime.

Switch off your phone at least an hour before going to bed. Very clever psychologists have designed the apps on your phone to attract your attention, wiring them into the dopamine centres of the brain. Switch off and let your brain relax.

Exercise earlier in the day is helpful for sleep. But exercising in the hour or two before bedtime might make it more difficult to get to sleep, so time your workout to help you get to sleep.

As well as caffeine, it's best to avoid eating late-night snacks, particularly any that are sugary. The glucose rush will act to hinder sleep.

The body is set to the natural day-night cycle, so ensuring your bedroom is properly dark will help sleep, as will reducing the levels of ambient light in the hour or two before bedtime. Also, make sure that your bedroom is not too warm: try to make sure it is cooler than the main living areas in your home.

Sweet dreams!

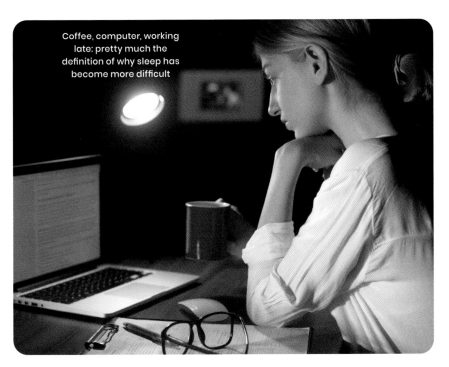

Coffee, computer, working late: pretty much the definition of why sleep has become more difficult

ANTI-INFLAMMATORY EXERCISE

Introduce some of these forms of exercise into your week to help reduce and relieve the symptoms of inflammation

O ne of the biggest lifestyle changes that you can make to improve inflammation is to make sure that you're doing enough exercise. Exercise helps you to get stronger and fitter, improves your heart health, builds muscles and bones, and can have a great effect on your mental health. It's well known that being physically inactive can increase the risk for things like type 2 diabetes, cardiovascular disease, dementia and some cancers. Those who are inactive are more likely to suffer from chronic inflammation, and find it harder to recover from acute inflammation too.

It's thought that when we exercise, we release certain cells into the body that have an anti-inflammatory effect. Plus, exercise helps us to maintain a healthy bodyweight and can reduce stress, both of which can also help to protect us against inflammation. Exercise can improve your sleep too, but be wary of working out too close to bedtime.

It's important to note that too much exercise at too high an intensity can actually have the opposite effect and can cause higher levels of inflammation. This can make us more susceptible to infection and illness – pro-level athletes, for example, may suffer from supressed immunity. It's important to exercise regularly, at a moderate intensity, and build in adequate rest days to make sure that you reap the benefits.

It doesn't really matter what kind of exercise you do – if it's something that you enjoy, then you're more likely to stick to it. Anything that gets your heart rate up is a great way of exercising your heart. Just make sure that you also do something to help your strength, and something to help your mobility and flexibility to balance all of your body's needs. If you do start to feel in pain or fatigued, then take some extra rest. This is a lifestyle, not a quick fix, so learn to listen to what your body needs.

Over these pages, we will look at six different types of exercise that you can try, known for their anti-inflammatory effects. We're all different, so it might take a little trial and error to work out what's right for you and your body. If you exercise already, then you may want to introduce some new forms of exercise to complement your existing routine. If you have an existing health condition, you may need to consult with your doctor before trying anything new.

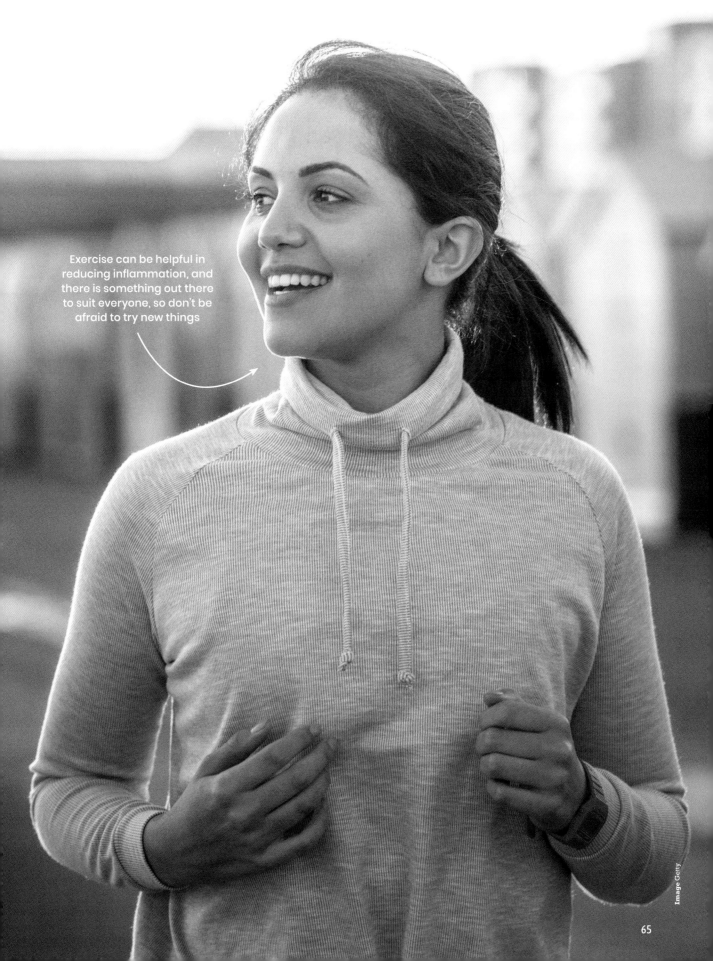

Exercise can be helpful in reducing inflammation, and there is something out there to suit everyone, so don't be afraid to try new things

Image Getty

65

1 WALKING

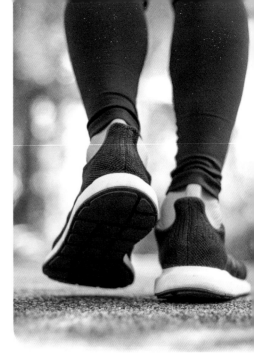

One of the simplest, but still effective, ways to manage inflammation is to go for a walk. It's low impact, inexpensive and accessible, but often overlooked as 'just walking'. For those who are new to exercise, it's a great way to introduce some cardiovascular work, and it's easy to progress as you get fitter. For those who already exercise, adding walking in on your rest days can help your body to recover and relax at a lower intensity. For the biggest benefits, do your walk outside, as being out in nature can also help with inflammation. You also need to consider your pace – you want to be walking briskly, so that your heart rate is elevated to around 60% of your maximum to get the greatest effect. It doesn't have to be a long walk though; one study* had participants walking on a treadmill at a moderate pace for just 20 minutes, which was enough to reduce inflammatory markers in the body. If you find it hard to get your heart rate up adequately when walking, then try adding in some hills to boost the challenge or extend the duration over time.

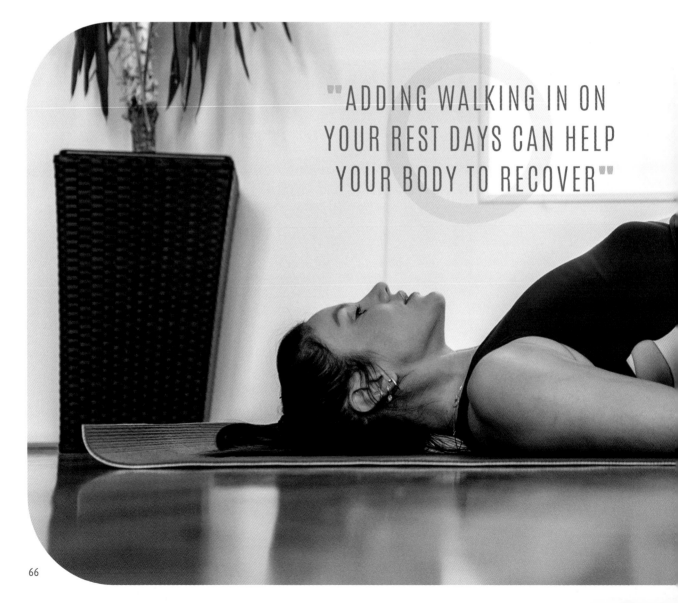

"ADDING WALKING IN ON YOUR REST DAYS CAN HELP YOUR BODY TO RECOVER"

② SIMPLE YOGA ROUTINE

Yoga is great for reducing inflammation, while building strength and flexibility. Try practising these three poses every day to help with chronic inflammation

① Supine Twist

Lie on your back, with your knees bent and feet on the floor. Open your arms out to your side in a 't' shape, then lift your knees up to your chest. Drop your knees to one side, turning your head in the opposite direction. Stay in this position, breathing deeply, for around 30-60 seconds, then repeat on the other side. This pose is great for digestive inflammation.

② Child's Pose

This rest position is perfect for relieving inflammation thanks to the slight inversion created with your head being lower than your hips. Start on your knees, with your thighs and feet together. Lower your bottom to your feet, and stretch your arms out in front of you, resting your forehead on the floor.

③ Bridge Pose

Lie on your back and bend your knees, with your feet firmly on the floor and your arms by your side, with your hands on the mat. Lift your hips up so that you're resting on the top of your back (not your neck) and hold for five deep breaths. This beginner's pose opens up the chest and can help increase blood flow and reduce inflammation in the body.

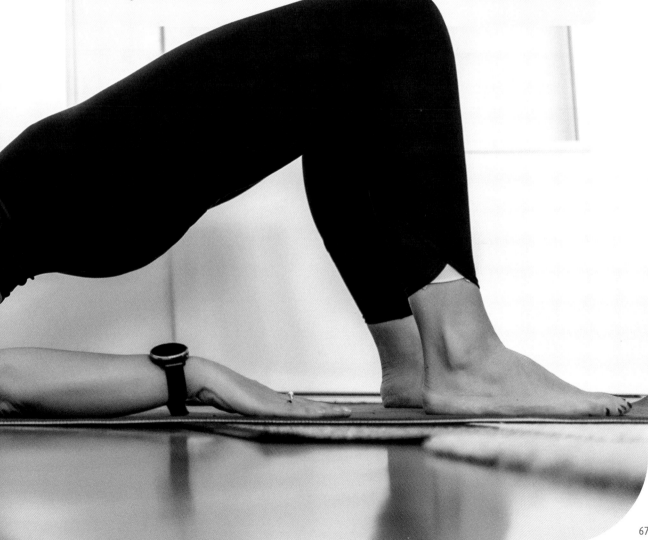

Images Getty. *Stoyan Dimitrov, et al. Inflammation and exercise: Inhibition of monocyte intracellular TNF production by acute exercise via β2-adrenergic activation. Brain, Behaviour & Immunity. 2017

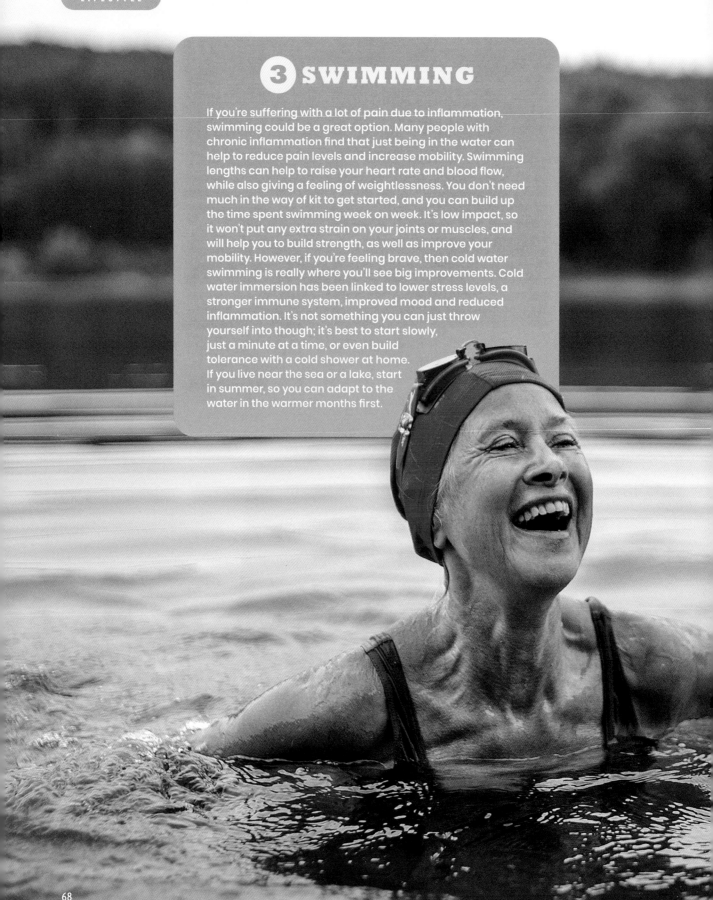

③ SWIMMING

If you're suffering with a lot of pain due to inflammation, swimming could be a great option. Many people with chronic inflammation find that just being in the water can help to reduce pain levels and increase mobility. Swimming lengths can help to raise your heart rate and blood flow, while also giving a feeling of weightlessness. You don't need much in the way of kit to get started, and you can build up the time spent swimming week on week. It's low impact, so it won't put any extra strain on your joints or muscles, and will help you to build strength, as well as improve your mobility. However, if you're feeling brave, then cold water swimming is really where you'll see big improvements. Cold water immersion has been linked to lower stress levels, a stronger immune system, improved mood and reduced inflammation. It's not something you can just throw yourself into though; it's best to start slowly, just a minute at a time, or even build tolerance with a cold shower at home. If you live near the sea or a lake, start in summer, so you can adapt to the water in the warmer months first.

4 BASIC BODYWEIGHT MOVES

Bodyweight exercise is perfect if you're new to strength work. It can improve your heart health, build your strength and boost your bones, Try this simple five-move routine a couple of times a week. Start off by doing each exercise for 30 seconds, resting for 30 seconds in between moves, and repeating the whole circuit three to five times. As you get fitter you can increase the time on each exercise or the number of circuits. We've suggested a few adaptions for each move too.

1 Squat
You can also try a wall squat, or practise standing up from a chair and sitting back down again.

2 Elbow plank
You can hold this on your knees rather than your feet.

3 Jumping jacks
If jumping is too much for your joints, then you can step out to each side instead.

4 Push-up
Start on your knees and progress to your feet. You can also try a standing push-up against a wall to begin with.

5 Bird dog
Start on all fours, then lift one arm and the opposite leg, hold, then swap sides. You could try doing one limb at a time, rather than an arm and a leg.

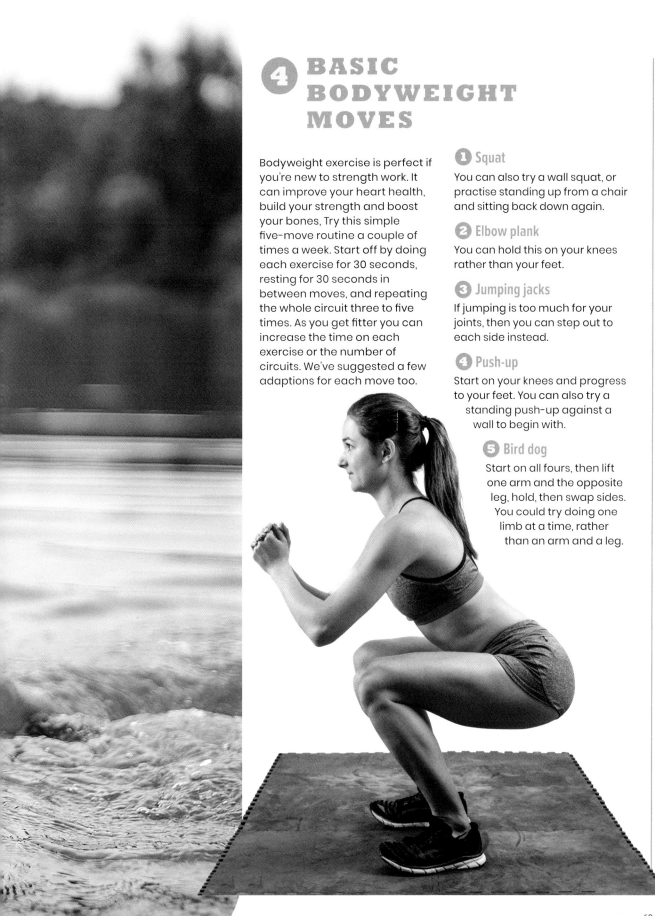

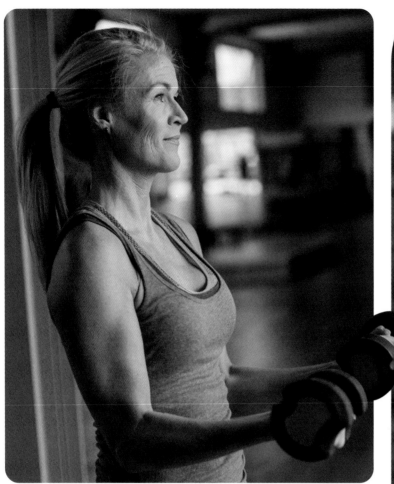

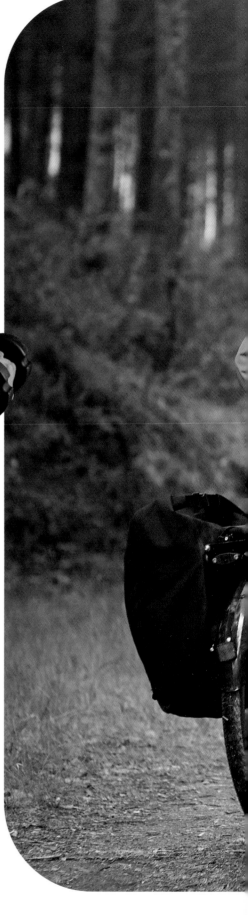

⑤ RESISTANCE TRAINING

Introducing some weights into your workouts can help to boost the anti-inflammatory effects of exercise. While many of the studies around inflammation and exercise focus on cardiovascular and endurance sport, there are huge benefits to building resistance training into your exercise routine. The NHS in England suggests at least two days a week should include strength exercises that work all the major muscle groups, which is the same as that recommended by the Center for Disease Control and Prevention in the USA. This can be bodyweight work (see 4), but adding weights for extra resistance can boost the benefits further. One review** suggests that adherence to a resistance training program long term could be an effective way to prevent or delay inflammatory chronic diseases. Try adding light weights to your bodyweight exercises, or join a class that uses weights. It's important to get some advice on technique to ensure you're lifting weights correctly so that you don't injure yourself. It's worth the effort though, as resistance training has been shown to decrease pro-inflammatory markers and improve chronic inflammation.

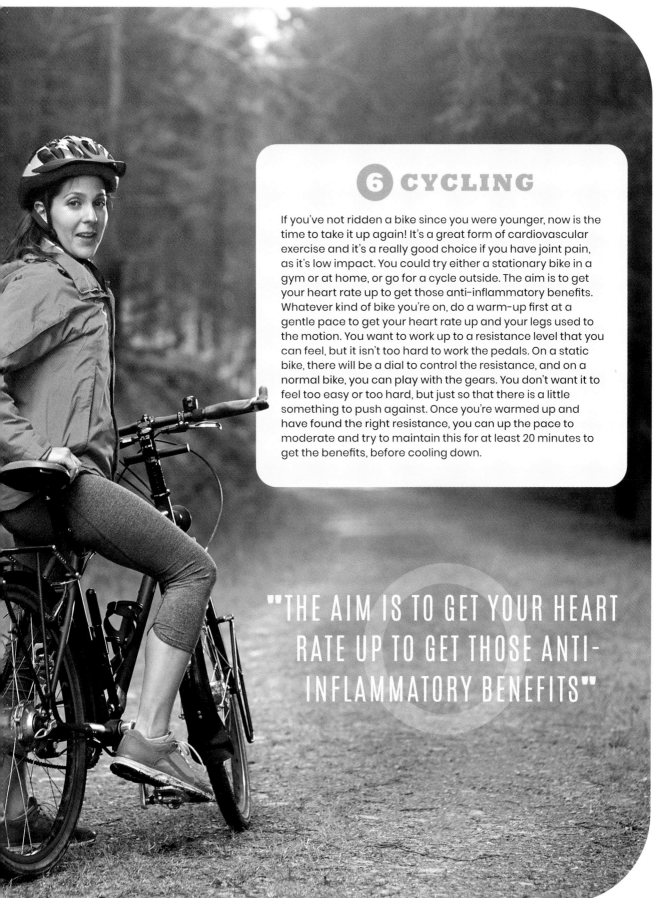

6 CYCLING

If you've not ridden a bike since you were younger, now is the time to take it up again! It's a great form of cardiovascular exercise and it's a really good choice if you have joint pain, as it's low impact. You could try either a stationary bike in a gym or at home, or go for a cycle outside. The aim is to get your heart rate up to get those anti-inflammatory benefits. Whatever kind of bike you're on, do a warm-up first at a gentle pace to get your heart rate up and your legs used to the motion. You want to work up to a resistance level that you can feel, but it isn't too hard to work the pedals. On a static bike, there will be a dial to control the resistance, and on a normal bike, you can play with the gears. You don't want it to feel too easy or too hard, but just so that there is a little something to push against. Once you're warmed up and have found the right resistance, you can up the pace to moderate and try to maintain this for at least 20 minutes to get the benefits, before cooling down.

"THE AIM IS TO GET YOUR HEART RATE UP TO GET THOSE ANTI-INFLAMMATORY BENEFITS"

Images Getty. **Calle MC, Fernandez ML. Effects of resistance training on the inflammatory response. Nutr Res Pract 2010

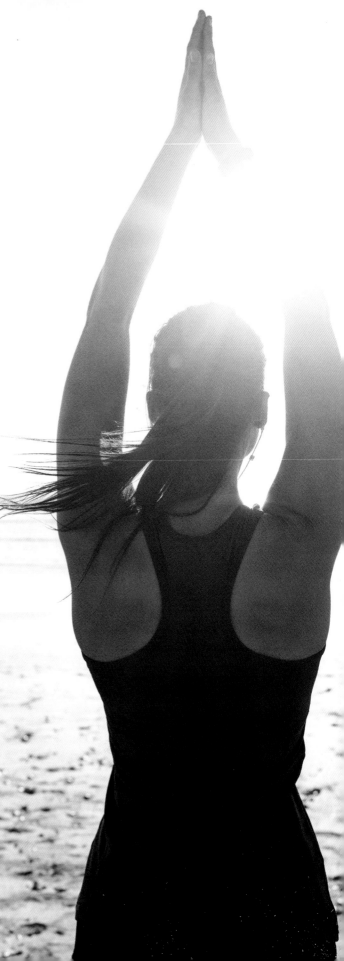

LESS PAIN, MORE GAIN!

You'll be pleased to hear that gentler exercise is good for you. Here's how to reap the benefits...

Take a look at the class list for most gyms and you can expect to see promises to "make you sweat" and "push you to the max". So it would be easy to think that hard and fast exercise is the only way to see changes.

While the ability to get your heart rate soaring is what gives high-intensity training its magical calorie-burning effect, that same intensity can also be its downfall. 'As your body starts to tire during a session, it will try to find easier ways to complete the moves,' explains Matt Harras, a group exercise manager for Virgin Active. 'You might start to rely on momentum (swinging a dumbbell instead of lifting with control), or try to switch the effort to other parts of the body, losing form.' This loss of form can reduce the effectiveness of the exercise. 'You can do 100 burpees but if you're not keeping form you won't see results. In that respect, slower and more controlled moves can actually be more beneficial.'

'It's a myth that you need to be huffing and puffing to see results,' says Niki Rein, founder of Barrecore. 'There are lots of different ways to get the same outcome. Resistance training can actually bring you further, faster than high-intensity cardio. It stimulates mitochondrial production – organisms that help create energy and melt fat. So as well as burning calories in class, you'll burn even more over the next three to four days.'

High-intensity exercise can also put pressure on joints, increase risk of injury and, when overdone, play havoc with our levels of the stress hormone cortisol. 'Too much HIIT (high intensity interval training) also puts pressure on the immune system as the body doesn't get a chance to recover,' reveals Matt. Take the pace down a few notches and you can turn those risk factors on their head. Low-intensity exercise helps protect joints and has been shown to reduce the level of stress hormones. Allow us to introduce you to some gentler but just as effective alternatives.

MAKE IT EASY ON YOURSELF

Train smarter instead of harder with these clever swaps

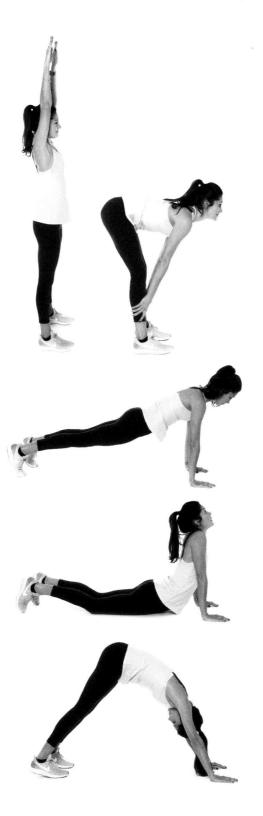

Swap burpees for sun salutations

///////////////////////////////

'Like a burpee but slower and with more control, which means you're holding your body weight for longer and focusing more on strength,' says Matt.

1 Stand with your feet hip-width apart. Stretch your arms up, then forwards and down towards your toes, keeping your back as flat as possible. Place your palms or fingertips on the floor in front of you (or on your ankles/shins), lift your head and hold for 10 seconds.

2 Plant your hands on the floor, walk your feet back into a plank position and hold for 10 seconds.

3 Slowly lower your knees, chest and chin towards the floor, with your body straight. Hover just above the floor for 10 seconds.

4 Drop your hips to the floor, straighten your arms and look up (upward-facing dog). Hold for 10 seconds.

5 Pushing into your palms, straighten your legs, raising your hips into the air and drop your head (downward-facing dog). Hold for 10 seconds.

6 Walk your feet back to your hands and slowly roll back up to standing.

7 Pause for 10 seconds then repeat the sequence four to five times.

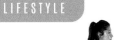

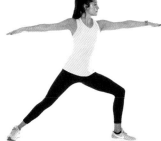

Swap jumping lunge for warrior pose

//////////////////

Jumping lunges are a great leg toner but can be hard on the knees. Matt suggests the warrior pose as a gentle alternative.

1 Stand with your feet wider than hip-width apart, arms straight out to the side at shoulder height, palms down. Turn the right foot out and bend the right knee until your thigh is parallel with the floor, making sure your knee doesn't go past your toes. Hold for 10 breaths.

2 Return to the centre and repeat on the other side. Repeat the sequence 3 times.

Swap press-ups for plank

//////////////////

'A press-up just works arms and chest – there's no time for your back muscles or core to develop,' says Paulo Pacifici, founder of the Ady Centre and DeRose Method teacher. 'Hold the plank position and you work the entire body.'

1 Start on all fours with your hands directly under your shoulders. Step your feet back and tuck your toes. Your body should form a straight line from the top of your head to your heels. Look down at the floor.

2 Hold for 45 seconds, building to 2 minutes. Focus on taking deep abdominal breaths through your nostrils.

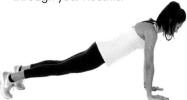

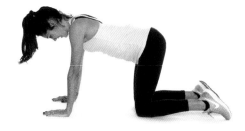

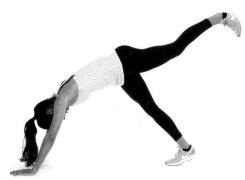

Swap mountain climbers for one-legged down dog

//////////////////////////

'It works the same muscle groups as mountain climbers but the slower pace should help you maintain stability and form, and increase the time under tension for your muscles, maximising results,' says Matt.

1 Start on all fours with your wrists directly under your shoulders and knees under your hips. Spread your fingers, tuck your toes and straighten your arms and legs, raising your hip into the air without locking your knees.

2 Step your feet together then lift your right leg into the air, flexing your foot.

3 Bring your knee in towards the chest and slowly extend back out. Repeat 10 times before switching to the other side. Repeat the sequence 3 times on each side.

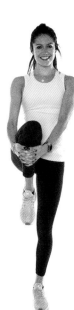

Swap high knees for holding leg pose

//////////////////////

Give high knees a clever makeover with this full-body workout from Paulo, which also improves balance.

1 Stand with your legs hip-width apart, arms by your side. Take a deep breath in and, on the exhale, lift your right knee towards your chest, as close as you can without bending your back. For more of a challenge, raise both arms above your head.

2 Hold for as long as possible, building up to one minute. Breathe through your nostrils and into your abdomen. Inhale as you lower your arm and leg then repeat on the other side.

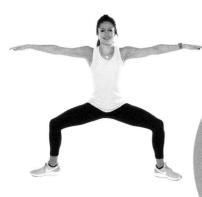

Swap squat jump for wide plie with pulse

///////////////

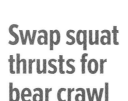
You won't be huffing and puffing but you'll feel the deep burning sensation, which is where the results are,' says Niki.

1. Stand with your legs wider than your hips, feet in a natural turn out. Lower your hips so your thighs are parallel to the floor, and hold your arms straight out at shoulder height (T position).

2. Bend your knees so your hips drop slightly lower than knee height or as low as possible without your knees buckling, raising your arms over your head. Lift your hips up a couple of inches, moving your arms back to the T position. Keep a neutral spine and your knees over your toes. Gently pulse up and down. Repeat 20 times slowly then 20 times at a faster, one-count rate.

3. Finish by holding in the lowest position for 15 seconds.

Swap squat thrusts for bear crawl

///////////////

Feel exhausted just thinking about squat thrusts? Try a bear crawl instead. 'It's a full-body exercise that will sculpt your shoulders and fire up your quads and glutes,' says Matt. 'Plus it's hard to get wrong.'

1. Crouch down with your hands on the floor, shoulder-width apart, hips in the air and eyes forward.

2. Crawl forward with your right hand and left leg then your left hand and right leg. Go forward five paces then back five paces. Repeat three times.

Swap sit ups/ crunches for dead bug

///////////////

'It's one of the simplest, most effective exercises to strengthen and tone your core,' says Matt.

1. Lie on your back, arms and thighs straight up to the ceiling, but with your knees bent to form a table top with your shins.

2. Engage the core to avoid rocking and slowly lower your right arm behind you while straightening and lowering your left leg. Tap the floor with your heel and hand then slowly move back to the start position before repeating with the other arm and leg. Repeat 20 times, 10 on each side. Rest for 30 seconds, then repeat.

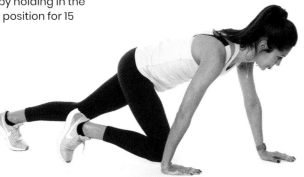

Images Anne Marie Bickerton, Getty Images

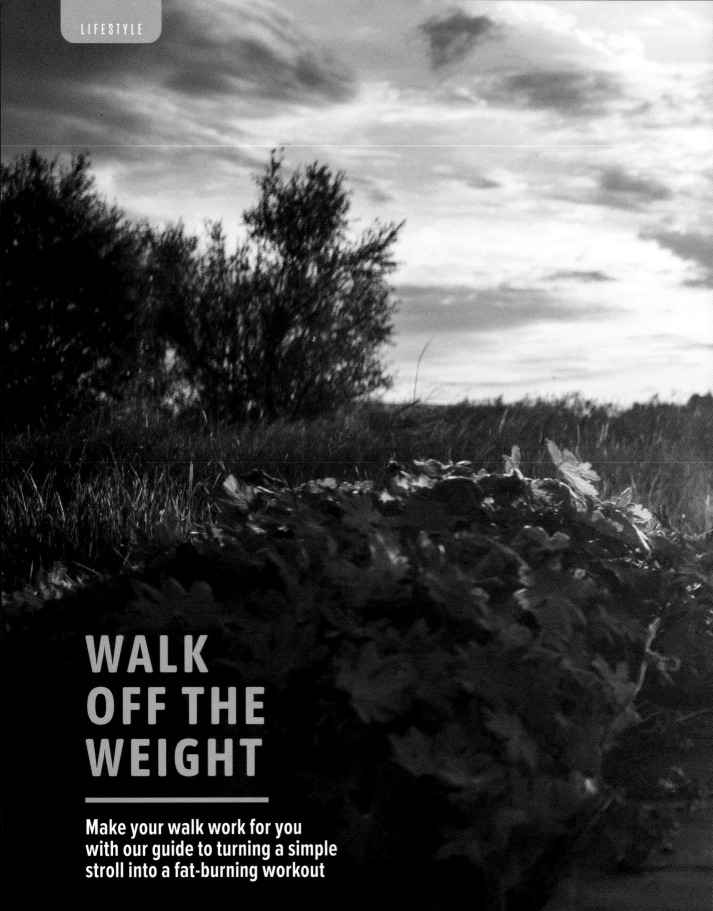

WALK OFF THE WEIGHT

Make your walk work for you with our guide to turning a simple stroll into a fat-burning workout

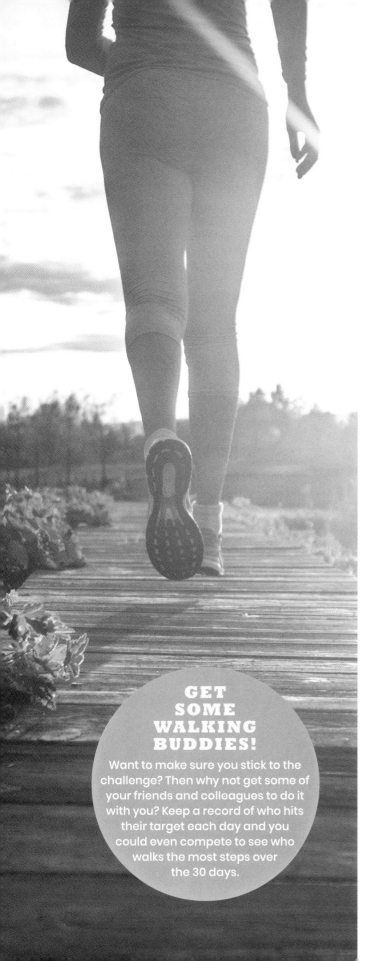

When we think of walking as exercise, it's usually more of a leisurely stroll or aiming for those coveted 10,000 steps a day. But walking is so much more than going from A to B, and when you do it properly, incorporating different paces, speeds and even elements such as lunges and squats, it can be a way to exercise that you hadn't thought of and helps the pounds fall away.

Walking is free and good for our health. The UK even has a National Walking Month in May, organised by the British Heart Foundation (**bhf.org.uk**). Just 30 minutes of exercise, including walking, five times a week reduces the risk of cardiovascular disease, cancer and type 2 diabetes, and could help relieve symptoms of depression. Plus, walking boosts circulation, making your skin look fresher and younger too.

Follow our plan and you'll be in shape within 30 days and singing the praises of walking to everyone you meet.

Your trainers

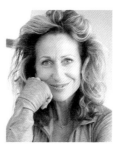 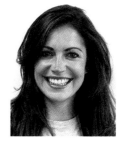

Joanna Hall (**joannahall.com**), creator of the Walkactive technique

Lucy Gornall, Freelance fitness writer and personal trainer

The challenge on the following pages is all about fitting extra activity into your busy day, and it's very simple.

There are three levels. Choose yours using the test on the next page, then follow the targets on the grid on the following page. If you find that your level is too easy, switch to a more advanced one – the key thing is the consistency of your efforts.

Do the daily walks in increments and the weekly walks when you can fit them in (for example, at the weekend – see over the page for details).

GET SOME WALKING BUDDIES!

Want to make sure you stick to the challenge? Then why not get some of your friends and colleagues to do it with you? Keep a record of who hits their target each day and you could even compete to see who walks the most steps over the 30 days.

THE 30-DAY CHALLENGE

Take the test

The amount of physical movement you do each day, without long periods of sitting, has the greatest impact on your health and fitness. You can track this by counting steps. Before you start the challenge, use a pedometer to record the number of steps you take for three consecutive days, then divide the total by three.

- If your daily average is less than 5,000, opt for the Novice Level.
- If your daily average is between 5,000 and 7,500, go for the Intermediate Level.
- If your daily average is 7,500+, choose the Whizz Level.

Now add in your weekend walks

Twice a week, do two brisk walks. Each should take 10-15 minutes, building up to 20-25 minutes.
Novice: 1,200-1,500 steps
Intermediate: 1,500 steps
Whizz: 1,700 steps

Days 8-14

Novice: 1,500-1,800 steps; Intermediate: 1,700 steps; Whizz: 1,800 steps

Days 15-22

Novice: 1,800 steps; Intermediate: 2,000 steps; Whizz: 2,500 steps

Days 23-30

Novice: 2,000 steps; Intermediate: 2,500 steps; Whizz: 3,000 steps

Get kitted out

Wearing the right kit will help you to focus on your walking journey…

- **Hike tights**
Sherpa Kalpana Hike Tight, **sherpaadventuregear.co.uk**. Every item you buy funds a school day for a child in Nepal.

- **Phone friend**
Freetrain V1 phone holder, **freetrain.co.uk**. Track those steps and free your arms.

- **Handy bag**
Quecchua Nature walking rucksack, **decathlon.co.uk**. An absolute steal!

- **Super shoe**
Columbia SH/FT OutDry mid shoe, **columbia sportswear.co.uk**. Special cushioning technology in the sole makes this a lightweight winner.

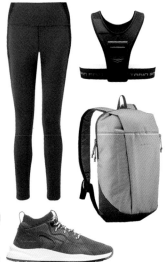

MAKE IT HARDER

If you really want to make your workout harder, Lucy recommends pausing your walk at every 1,000 steps and aiming for either 10 (Novice), 20 (Intermediate) or 30 (Whizz) repetitions of the below.

Curtsy lunge (split the rep count between each leg).Feet shoulder-width apart, step your left leg behind you and to the right. Bend both knees so you're in a curtsy position. From here, jump to the side to switch the position of your legs, ending in a curtsy lunge with leg positions reversed.

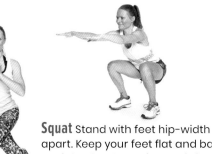

Squat Stand with feet hip-width apart. Keep your feet flat and back straight, then lower into a sitting position. Lift your arms out in front of you to balance. Hold for 3 seconds, push your heels into the floor and drive up to standing.

Eagle Squat Start with your legs together. Lift your right leg over your left leg, so they're crossed. Interlink your arms so your right elbow is underneath your left, palms touching. Squat down, hold for 3 seconds, switch sides and repeat.

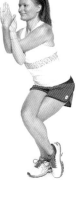

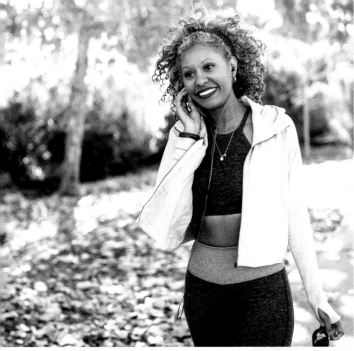

Day 1
Novice
5,000 steps
Intermediate
7,000 steps
Whizz
7,500 steps

Day 2
Novice
5,000 steps
Intermediate
7,000 steps
Whizz
7,500 steps

Day 3
Novice
5,000 steps
Intermediate
7,000 steps
Whizz
7,500 steps

Day 4
Novice
5,000 steps
Intermediate
7,000 steps
Whizz
7,500 steps

Day 5
Novice
5,000 steps
Intermediate
7,000 steps
Whizz
7,500 steps

Day 6
Novice
5,000 steps
Intermediate
7,000 steps
Whizz
7,500 steps

Day 7
Novice
5,000 steps
Intermediate
7,000 steps
Whizz
7,500 steps

Day 8
Novice
5,550 steps
Intermediate
7,500 steps
Whizz
8,000 steps

Day 9
Novice
5,550 steps
Intermediate
7,500 steps
Whizz
8,000 steps

Day 10
Novice
5,550 steps
Intermediate
7,500 steps
Whizz
8,000 steps

Day 11
Novice
5,550 steps
Intermediate
7,500 steps
Whizz
8,000 steps

Day 12
Novice
5,550 steps
Intermediate
7,500 steps
Whizz
8,000 steps

Day 13
Novice
5,550 steps
Intermediate
7,500 steps
Whizz
8,000 steps

Day 14
Novice
5,550 steps
Intermediate
7,500 steps
Whizz
8,000 steps

Day 15
Novice
6,000 steps
Intermediate
8,000 steps
Whizz
9,000 steps

Day 16
Novice
6,000 steps
Intermediate
8,000 steps
Whizz
9,000 steps

Day 17
Novice
6,000 steps
Intermediate
8,000 steps
Whizz
9,000 steps

Day 18
Novice
6,000 steps
Intermediate
8,000 steps
Whizz
9,000 steps

Day 19
Novice
6,000 steps
Intermediate
8,000 steps
Whizz
9,000 steps

Day 20
Novice
6,000 steps
Intermediate
8,000 steps
Whizz
9,000 steps

Day 21
Novice
6,000 steps
Intermediate
8,000 steps
Whizz
9,000 steps

Day 22
Novice
6,000 steps
Intermediate
8,000 steps
Whizz
9,000 steps

Day 23
Days 23–30 targets
Novice
51,500 steps
Intermediate
68,000 steps
Whizz
80,000 steps

Day 24
Novice
6,500 steps
Intermediate
8,500 steps
Whizz
10,000 steps

Day 25
Novice
6,500 steps
Intermediate
8,500 steps
Whizz
10,000 steps

Day 26
Novice
6,500 steps
Intermediate
8,500 steps
Whizz
10,000 steps

Day 27
Novice
6,500 steps
Intermediate
8,500 steps
Whizz
10,000 steps

Day 28
Novice
6,500 steps
Intermediate
8,500 steps
Whizz
10,000 steps

Day 29
Novice
6,500 steps
Intermediate
8,500 steps
Whizz
10,000 steps

Day 30
Novice
6,500 steps
Intermediate
8,500 steps
Whizz
10,000 steps

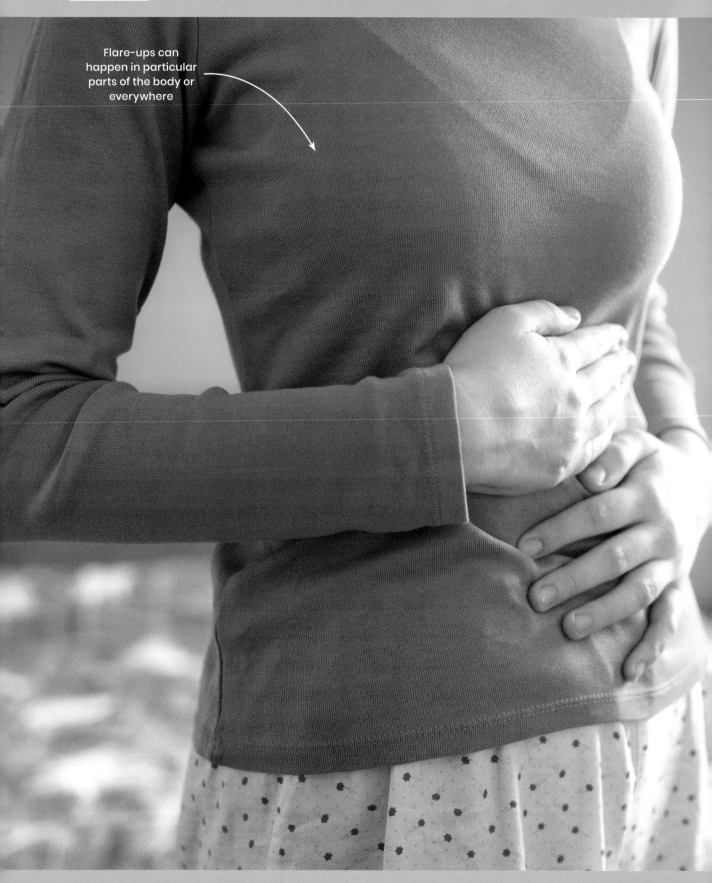

Flare-ups can happen in particular parts of the body or everywhere

HOW TO CALM
CHRONIC
INFLAMMATION

**SOME SIMPLE STRATEGIES TO HELP COPE WITH
FLARE-UPS OF CHRONIC INFLAMMATION**

Many of the conditions associated with chronic inflammation, such as arthritis, chronic pain and inflammatory bowel disease, are prone to sudden flare-ups when, often for no obvious reason, they suddenly become much worse. For people suffering from these conditions, these are difficult times, with no magic bullet solutions.

However, there are some strategies that might help to alleviate the symptoms. It's nevertheless the case that what is effective for one person might produce hardly any benefit for another. In large part, it's a case of experimenting, through trial and error, to find out what works for you. As such, it helps to have an array of options that you can try when the body feels like it catches fire.

There are two main avenues to explore apart from medication: what you eat and drink and what you do. Let's start with what you eat and drink.

Starting with drink, chronic inflammation is bound up with chronic stress in an unholy feedback loop. To cope with chronic stress we often resort to short-term fixes: an extra glass of wine, another cup of coffee, something sweet and fizzy to top up our energy or make us feel a bit better. Of these, the caffeine in coffee and, to a lesser extent tea, will stimulate a system that has become incapable of slowing down, wiring it up further and exacerbating inflammation. So cutting back, or cutting out, coffee and tea is one strategy to try, as is stopping fizzy, sugary drinks such as cola. With their high sugar content, fizzy drinks are instant energy fixes – exactly what we don't need when the body is already wired.

Unlike coffee and caffeinated drinks, alcohol is not a stimulant but rather a depressant. In very moderate amounts, it can possibly be helpful. But anything more than one glass of wine is likely to start causing problems to a stressed body. A hangover is the body having to deal with the toxic effects of too much alcohol, which will only make chronic inflammation worse. So better to cut down or cut out entirely during a flare-up.

As for what we do, gentle exercise will, in almost all cases, be beneficial. The human body is made to move and, in particular, to walk. Walking, and other forms of gentle exercise such as yoga, are all positively beneficial with virtually no downsides. More vigorous exercise may also work but will depend on the sort of flare-up that you are suffering from.

One of the key ways that exercise helps is that it makes it easier, afterwards, to sleep better. Along with exercise, a good night's sleep is the great healer. Inflammatory flare-ups can make it harder to sleep. Ensure a settled bedtime routine by avoiding caffeine and alcohol and switching off devices to get that healing, restful sleep.

We were made to walk and walking makes us feel better, even if help is needed

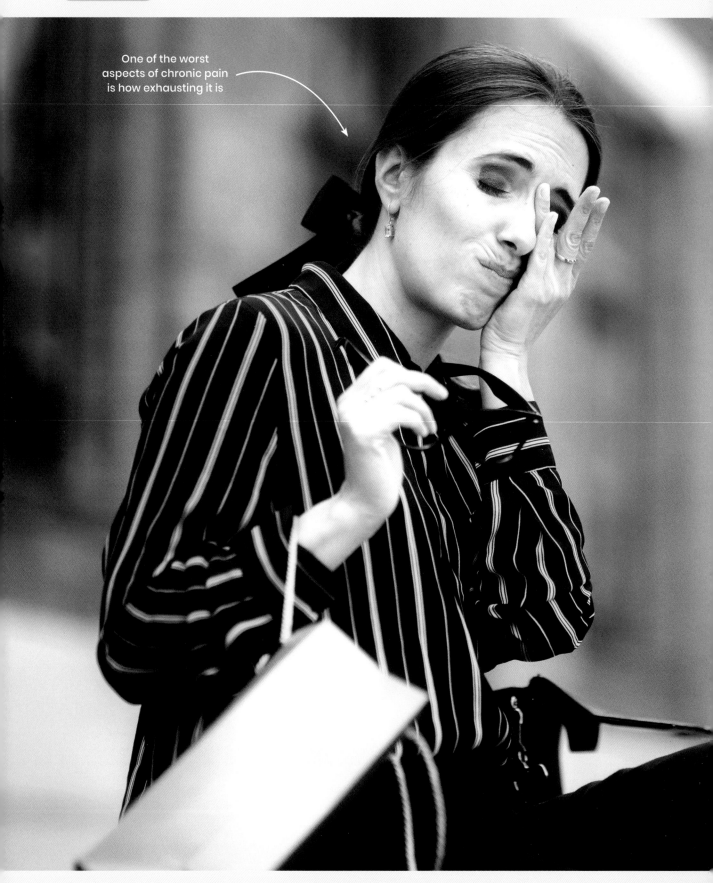

One of the worst aspects of chronic pain is how exhausting it is

There's no two ways about it: the diseases and conditions caused by chronic inflammation are horrible. Because chronic inflammation can affect every part of the body, as well as the mind, the conditions associated with it are many. And even with the best care and despite the sufferer doing everything 'right' to ameliorate their condition, it remains a heavy burden of ill health to bear.

In general, people suffering from chronic inflammation have spent a lot of time doing a huge amount of research on the subject. As such, few things are more irritating than some well-wisher chirping, "Have you tried mindfulness?" Yes, they have almost certainly tried mindfulness, along with a whole host of other strategies.

So, these ideas are offered as an aide memoire to people suffering from chronic inflammation and its associated conditions. You have most probably tried all of these before. But it's possible, amid the grind of dealing with a body that is playing up in this way, that you might have forgotten one or two of these possibilities. It's also true that what did not work at one point might work, under different conditions, today. So keep this as a checklist of things to try.

If you are under the care of a doctor, it's worth going to see him or her again for further advice. No, you won't be wasting their time: it's their job. Even if it's impossible to arrange an appointment, it's worth checking that you are carrying out all medical advice: it's all too easy to forget or skimp on something, which might be enough to exacerbate your inflammation.

For short term help, over-the-counter anti-inflammatory drugs such as ibuprofen might be helpful, or if the pain is localised it might be worth rubbing an ibuprofen gel into the area. Remember that you can't use NSAIDs if you're on steroid medication, however.

Gentle stretching might help. This doesn't have to be some contorted yoga pose but simply stretching and holding, for between two and five minutes, will sometimes help alleviate muscle pain. It's worth trying to hold the stretch for this longer time rather than just doing a ten-second stretch as it takes a while to overcome the body's stretch reflex and settle into the stretch.

Rest, exercise, particularly walking, and sleep are good for everyone and even more important for people suffering from chronic inflammation, as they allow the body to begin to unwind. Modern life makes all of these difficult, but if they can be integrated into your daily routine they should make a difference. Good luck!

"CHRONIC INFLAMMATION CAN AFFECT EVERY PART OF THE BODY"

Image Getty

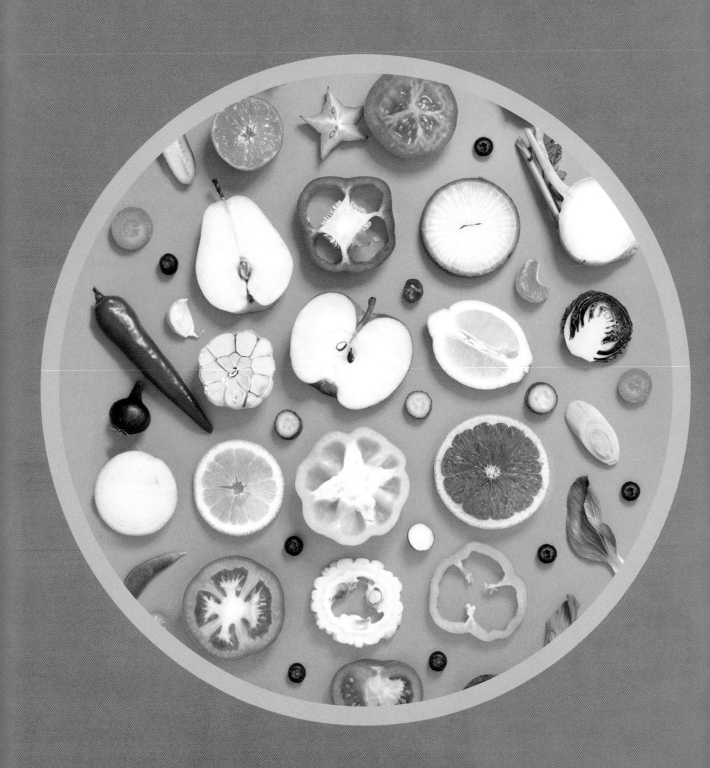

(3)

•••○

HEALTH

//

Learn about the role of gut health in chronic inflammation. Plus an in-depth guide to the best anti-inflammatory foods, and those you should minimise or avoid where possible.

TRUST YOUR GUT

When it comes to arming your body for the battle against inflammation, your gut is your most important ally. Here's how you can give it the tools it needs to keep you fighting fit

Despite its name, the gut (derived from the old English word 'guttas', meaning 'a channel') is a fascinating and integral part of the human body. Consisting of the colon, intestine and stomach, your gastrointestinal system is responsible for digesting what you consume, absorbing and redirecting the nutrients within it and getting rid of any waste through excretion. It is a busy department, with a direct line to your brain via the vagus nerve. This crucial link (known as the gut-brain axis) allows for the transmission of information from the gut to the brain that helps to regulate sleep, pain, mood, stress and – you guessed it – hunger.

Measuring around 1.5 metres in length, your large intestine is home to approximately 200 different species of fungi, bacteria and viruses that make up your gut microbiome. It is these clever little organisms (scientists estimate that your large intestine is home to about 39 trillion bacterial cells) that assist in turning what you eat into the nutrients that your body needs. An incredible 70–80 per cent of your immune cells are present in the gut, which is why improving your gut health is fundamental to supporting a robust immune system that is capable of dealing with the threat of inflammation effectively and efficiently when called upon.

However, enhancing your gut health isn't simply a question of sourcing good microorganisms. As with most things in life, a strong gut requires a balanced microbiome, and this is contingent upon various factors, your diet chief among them. Failing to eat a wide enough variety of fruit, vegetable and whole grains, not getting enough prebiotics and drinking too much alcohol can all contribute to creating an imbalance in your gut. In turn this can lead to a range of problems that can impact the immune system,

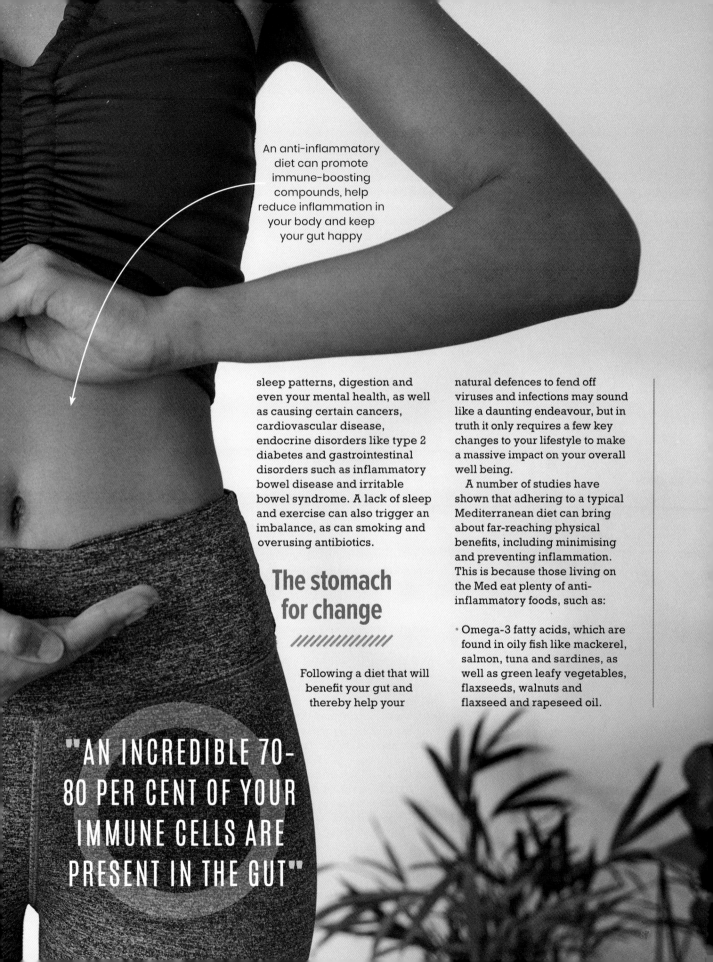

An anti-inflammatory diet can promote immune-boosting compounds, help reduce inflammation in your body and keep your gut happy

sleep patterns, digestion and even your mental health, as well as causing certain cancers, cardiovascular disease, endocrine disorders like type 2 diabetes and gastrointestinal disorders such as inflammatory bowel disease and irritable bowel syndrome. A lack of sleep and exercise can also trigger an imbalance, as can smoking and overusing antibiotics.

The stomach for change

//////////////

Following a diet that will benefit your gut and thereby help your

natural defences to fend off viruses and infections may sound like a daunting endeavour, but in truth it only requires a few key changes to your lifestyle to make a massive impact on your overall well being.

A number of studies have shown that adhering to a typical Mediterranean diet can bring about far-reaching physical benefits, including minimising and preventing inflammation. This is because those living on the Med eat plenty of anti-inflammatory foods, such as:

• Omega-3 fatty acids, which are found in oily fish like mackerel, salmon, tuna and sardines, as well as green leafy vegetables, flaxseeds, walnuts and flaxseed and rapeseed oil.

"AN INCREDIBLE 70–80 PER CENT OF YOUR IMMUNE CELLS ARE PRESENT IN THE GUT"

- Polyphenols, the plant chemicals found in apples, berries, citrus, soybeans and dark chocolate to name a few.
- Unsaturated fats, which come from seeds like sesame, pumpkin and flax, nuts including almonds, pecans and walnuts, and plant oils like olive, rapeseed and peanut.
- Fibre, which comes in the form of wholegrains like oats, barley and bran but also vegetables and fruits and in particular legumes.

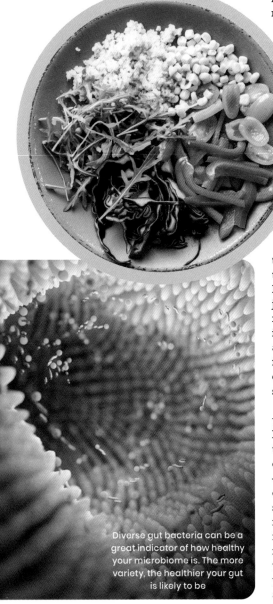

Diverse gut bacteria can be a great indicator of how healthy your microbiome is. The more variety, the healthier your gut is likely to be

Phytochemicals are yet another weapon in your arsenal against inflammation. Found in a wide variety of foods including tomatoes, broccoli, berries, pears, carrots and spinach, phytochemicals act as anti-inflammatory and antioxidant agents to help counteract the harmful effects of inflammation and bring down swelling throughout the body.

You don't necessarily need to strictly follow the Mediterranean menu, but one thing you should always be aiming to do is enjoy foods that are as close to their natural state as possible, in order to reap their full anti-inflammatory benefits.

Minimally processed and fresh foods retain their nutritional value and are free from the nasties that can impact your gut health, such as emulsifiers, artificial sweeteners and various additives.

Drinking plenty of water is another way to boost your gut health. This is because water assists in the breakdown of food, helping to absorb nutrients and increase the diversity of bacteria in the gut. It is also critical for lubricating our joints (60 per cent of your body is made up of water, and most of this is stored in connective tissue such as tendons and ligaments) and flushing out toxins that could otherwise trigger inflammation, such as gout.

Always keep in mind that when you are embracing a new diet it's best to start off slowly. Try to think of it more as a lifestyle change than "going on a diet" – gradually switch your meal choices from sugar- or salt-laden snacks poured from a packet to nourishing foods that originate from the ground. The more natural, colourful and varied your food, the better equipped your body will be to both fight and prevent inflammation.

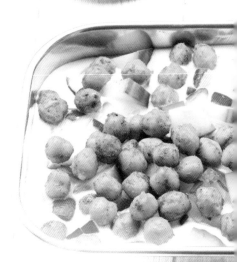

Make sure meals that fight inflammation and disease are on the menu! Foods rich in pro- and prebiotics like legumes and yoghurt are recommended daily

Research shows that various dietary patterns are linked to a lower risk of inflammation and that making certain dietary choices could further aid in the reduction of chronic inflammation in the body, which is linked to a vastly increased risk of stroke and developing diseases including Alzheimer's.

A mixed approach

Embracing an anti-inflammatory diet should go hand in hand with your lifestyle. Therefore, in addition to fueling your body with the optimum anti-inflammatory foods to keep your gut happy and your immune system ready, you will also need to ease lower levels of inflammation caused by other means.

A solid night's sleep is a good place to start, and by this we mean seven uninterrupted hours of slumber. While you're snoozing your body relaxes, including your blood vessels, and your blood pressure also drops. However, if

Images Getty

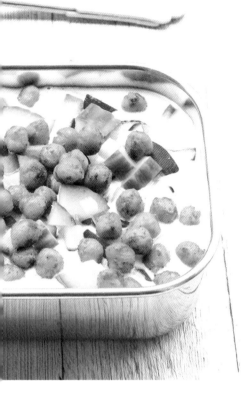

you're not getting enough shuteye your body doesn't get the chance to relax and recharge, meaning that your blood pressure doesn't decline. Studies suggest this can lead to cells present in the walls of your blood vessels initiating an inflammatory response.

Daily exercise is also integral to mitigating inflammation. You only need to exercise a little every day to help reduce the presence of pro-inflammatory cytokines such as tumour necrosis factor (TNF). This protein helps your body to heal by guiding inflammatory cells to the site of an injury, but too much of it can lead to negative inflammation. Thankfully research has shown that just 20 minutes of movement a day can lessen the amount of TNF your body produces, thereby easing the risk of inflammation.

Tackling stress is yet another way that you can ensure you are doing all you can to fight inflammation. When your body experiences stress your fight-or-flight response is triggered. Along with suppressing your immune system and flooding your body with adrenaline (in order to help you flee the perceived danger) your body also releases cytokines (like TNF). In normal circumstances these inflammatory warriors charge out, deal with the threat and withdraw, but if someone experiences chronic stress these inflammatory-causing cells can wreak havoc instead.

Thankfully there are several ways you can learn to cope with stress, including breathing exercises, yoga, walking the dog or talking to a friend or therapist. Whatever works for you, it's vital that you don't neglect your mental health as you pursue better physical health.

Don't keep the doctor away

////////////////

While the advantages of maintaining good gut health and eating plenty of anti-inflammatory foods are clear, it's important to remember that no diet is a cure for chronic or autoimmune conditions, and nor should any of the advice given in this book be viewed as a substitute for expert medical advice from your GP.

It's also worth noting that there may be certain foods that trigger inflammation specifically in your gut. If this is the case, keep a food diary and try eliminating these items or food groups from your diet and noting down any changes. Symptoms ranging from fatigue to irregular blood sugar levels and severe constipation can be linked to inflammation in your gut. Ultimately, if you have any worries about your gut health then speaking to a health professional or nutritionist is always recommended.

The fundamental goal of an anti-inflammatory lifestyle is simple – to lessen or, if possible, prevent inflammation in your body and thereby help you to minimise your risk of developing a whole host of ailments and diseases. So the next time you feel like reaching for a sugary treat or a fatty option on the menu, try to remember the importance of a happy gut in your quest against unwanted inflammation. Equally, be sure not to be too hard on yourself; taking gradual steps towards a healthier way of life is far more effective than punishing yourself in the short-term, a method that you will grow to resent and eventually discard. A balanced approach is the way to go.

Anti-inflammatory diets are often encouraged by health experts not just to combat inflammation but for general good health

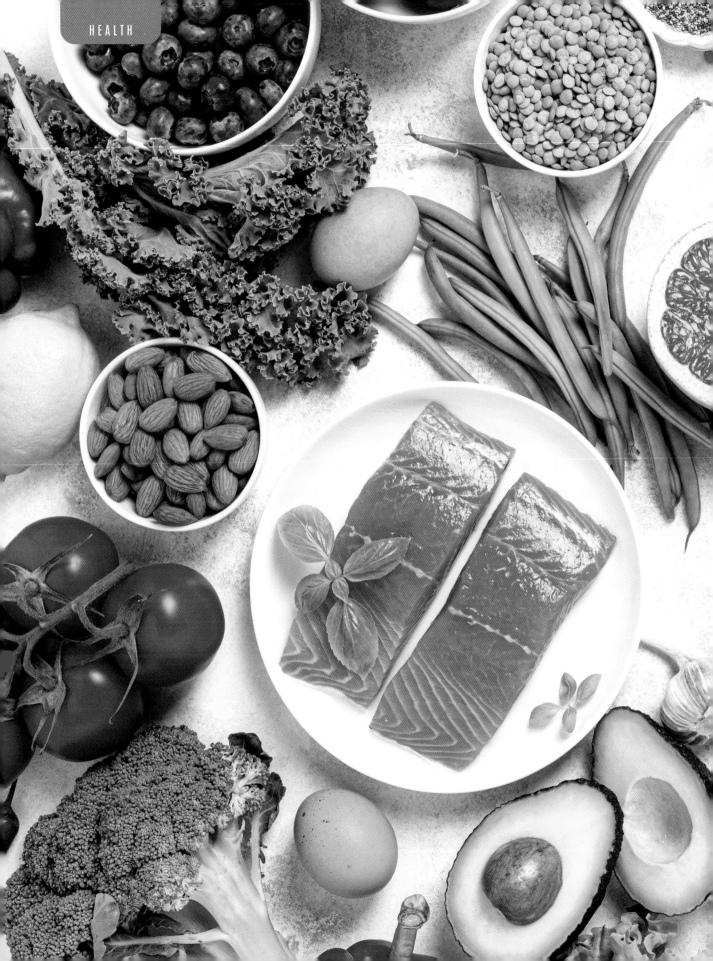

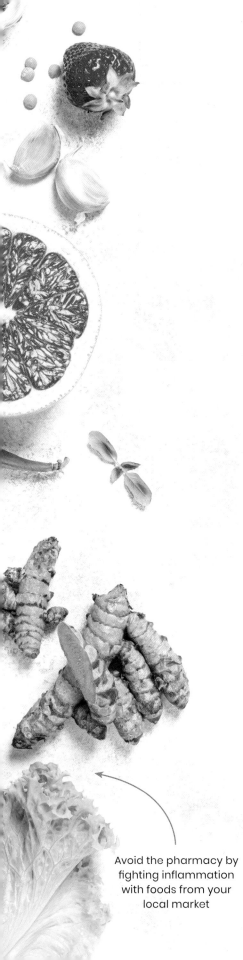

ANTI-INFLAMMATORY FOODS

Add these crucial ingredients to your arsenal in the battle to stave off the threat of inflammation and maintain a healthy lifestyle

Avoid the pharmacy by fighting inflammation with foods from your local market

We all know how important it is to take care of ourselves, but with people's lives busier than they've ever been, in a world where it seems like something is always demanding our attention, maintaining a healthy and balanced diet is easier said than done. Even so, we are blessed to live in a world with so much choice, particularly when it comes to fuelling our bodies and supporting our gut health. As the saying goes, you are what you eat, and choosing foods that are packed with antioxidants, minerals, phytonutrients and vitamins is absolutely crucial, especially if you want to keep inflammation at bay.

As with most things, when it comes to inflammation it is a question of balance. This is because there are certain types of inflammation, and these can be both detrimental and beneficial to the body.

Excessive inflammation can negatively affect the nervous system, joints and organs, thereby increasing the risk of various conditions including heart and bowel disease, high blood pressure and even depression. On the flip side, we also need inflammation in order for our bodies to heal. For example, when we have an infection, suffer an injury or experience trauma, the immune system responds by triggering what is known as acute inflammation in order to activate the healing process.

Certain foods can trigger negative inflammation. Processed meats, deep-fried foods, sugar-sweetened beverages, bread and pasta made with white flour, cookies, cakes, pies and foods high in added sugars or trans fats are definitely best avoided. The way in which we prepare our meals also has an effect, which is why stir frying, air frying and steaming have become increasingly popular.

Fortunately, there are plenty of tasty and healthy anti-inflammatory food options out there that can help to fight off the threat of inflammation and keep you feeling your very best. Here we will take a closer look at a range of anti-inflammatory options and find out why fresh and simple ingredients really are always the best additions to your shopping trolley.

Image Getty

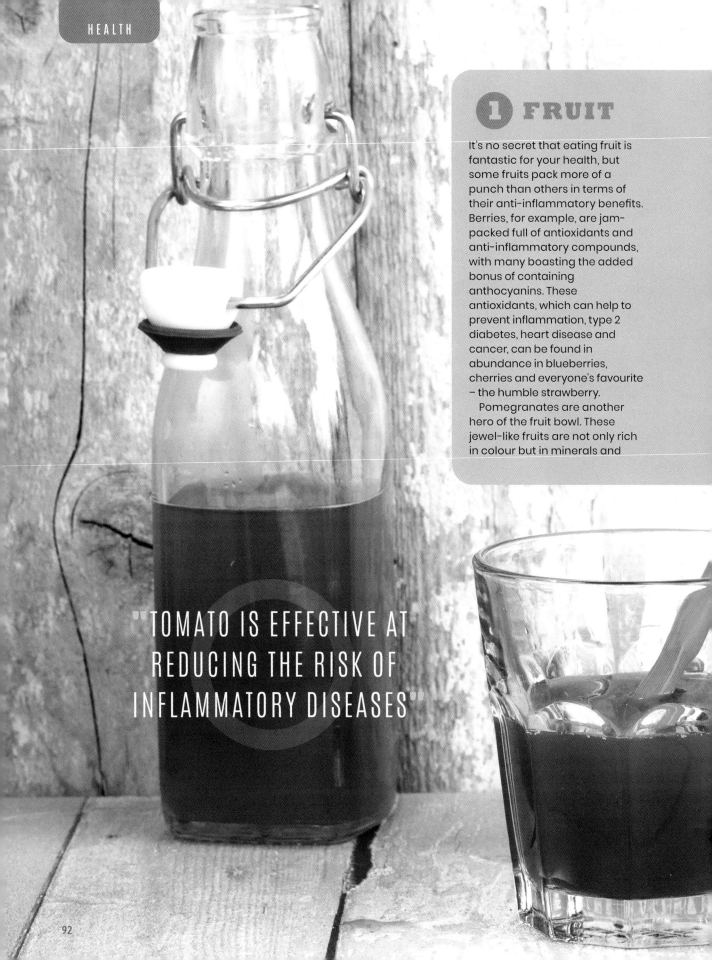

1 FRUIT

It's no secret that eating fruit is fantastic for your health, but some fruits pack more of a punch than others in terms of their anti-inflammatory benefits. Berries, for example, are jam-packed full of antioxidants and anti-inflammatory compounds, with many boasting the added bonus of containing anthocyanins. These antioxidants, which can help to prevent inflammation, type 2 diabetes, heart disease and cancer, can be found in abundance in blueberries, cherries and everyone's favourite – the humble strawberry.

Pomegranates are another hero of the fruit bowl. These jewel-like fruits are not only rich in colour but in minerals and

"TOMATO IS EFFECTIVE AT REDUCING THE RISK OF INFLAMMATORY DISEASES"

vitamins, boasting an additional antioxidant content that is three times higher than that found in either red wine or green tea. Pomegranates contain ellagitannins that when consumed act as antioxidants and help to reduce inflammation in the body.

This magic fruit, whether added to a savoury or sweet meal or juiced for a quick hit, can aid in protecting the brain against inflammation and oxidative stress, help the brain to recover from injury while also promoting optimal gut health.

Another big hitter is the good old tomato. Classified as a fruit because of its seeds, this household staple contains one of the richest sources of lycopene, which is a highly potent antioxidant and carotenoid. Possessing powerful anti-inflammatory properties, the tomato is effective at reducing the risk of inflammatory diseases (cooked tomatoes even more so), plus they have the added bonus of offering a good kick of vitamin C.

Red grapes are another great tool for combating inflammation due to their high content of anthocyanins and the pigment quercetin, which has antioxidant and anti-inflammatory properties. They also contain resveratrol, a chemical that hails from the polyphenol family and provides us with a host of health benefits, including improving the function of the blood vessels and protecting against heart inflammation. It can be found in red wine and grape juice too.

The real beauty of fresh fruit is that it's completely free from labels, meaning that it hasn't been tampered with or overprocessed. Including a variety of fruits in your daily diet (and experimenting with new ones when you get the chance to) is fundamental to good physical and mental health. By boosting our energy levels, lessening pain, soothing inflammation and enhancing mental clarity, fruit can play a critical role in ensuring that your body is absorbing a wealth of vital nutrients.

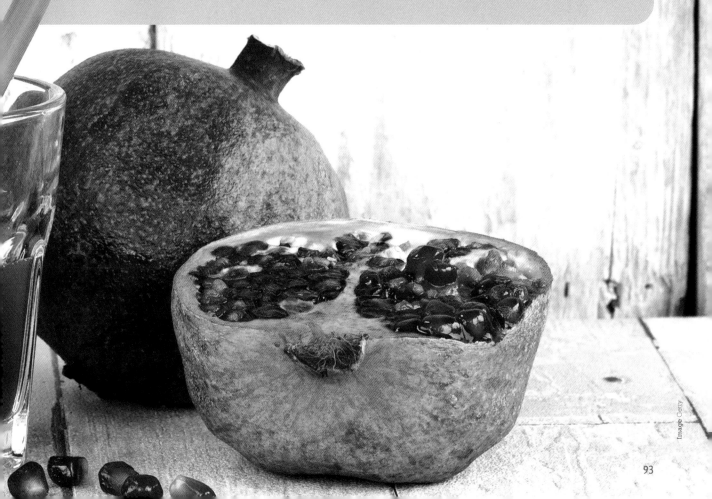

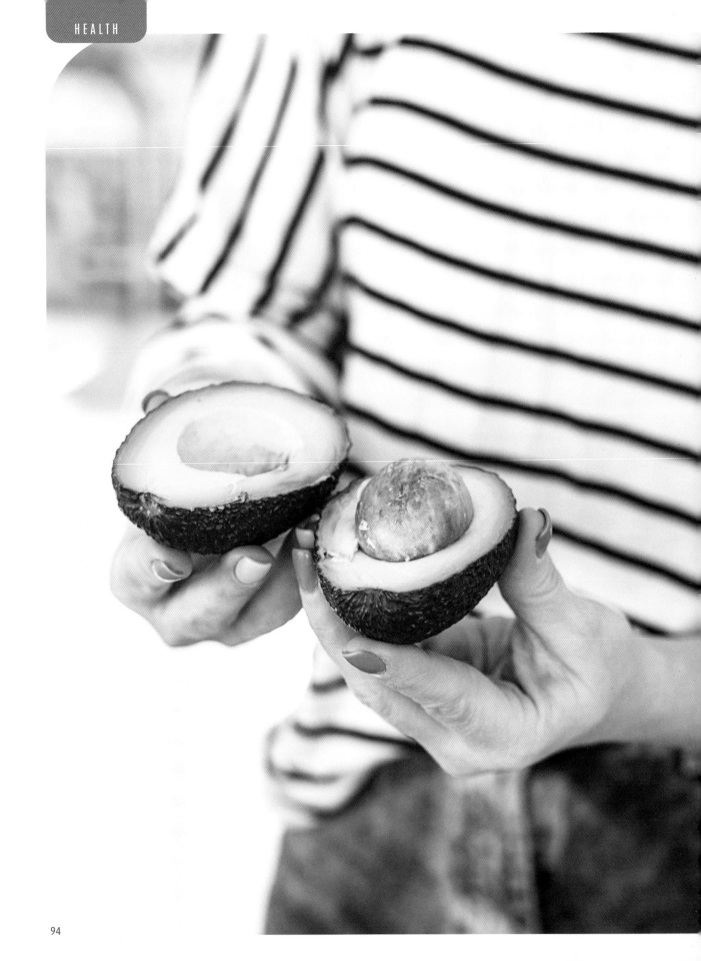

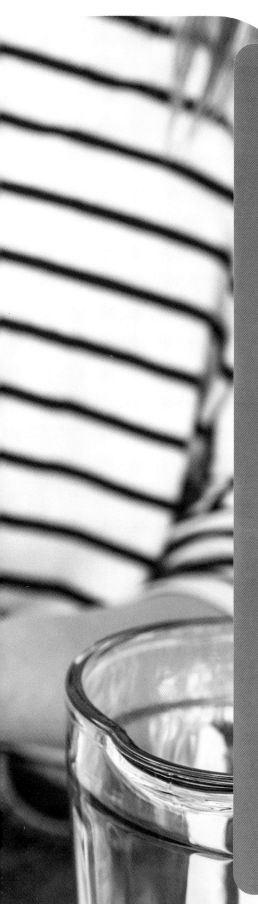

2 VEGETABLES

Defined by botanists as a fruit due to its single seed, the avocado is often thought of as a vegetable. One thing that can be agreed on, however, is that these pear-shaped beauties are an anti-inflammatory must. Home to carotenoids and tocopherols that reduce the risk of cancer, monounsaturated fats that lower cholesterol, fibre (which assists gut health), potassium and magnesium, this all-round superfood also contains linoleic and oleic acids. Studies have found that these acids can lessen the number of inflammatory cells in the wake of an injury and boost the healing process. Now all you have to do is figure out when it's ripe!

If you're not a fan of avocado on toast then drop one into a smoothie with some kale or green leafy vegetables (such as spinach) for a Popeye-approved hit of glucosinolates. With their anti-inflammatory effect on the body, glucosinolates are high in antioxidants and contain a protective compound found in plants called polyphenols that can fight neurodegenerative and cardiovascular diseases. Cruciferous vegetables like leafy greens, broccoli, spinach, cauliflower, sprouts and kale all contain polyphenols, and the latter is also naturally rich in sulforaphane. This is another powerful antioxidant that helps to reduce the levels of the molecules nuclear factor kappa B (NF-κB) and cytokines, and it is these that are responsible for creating inflammation.

By eating all the colours of the vegetable rainbow, you will help to maximise your vitamin and nutrient intake. Enjoy red bell peppers for a vitamin C and quercetin hit, chilli peppers for their ferulic and sinapic acid, and mushrooms for B vitamins, copper, selenium and ergothioneine, the antioxidant said to increase levels of the anti-inflammatory hormone adiponectin, which many people with type 2 diabetes cannot often produce enough of.

Root vegetables are also known to be effective when it comes to extinguishing inflammation. Due to their high content of the potent anti-inflammatory compound falcarindiol, raw carrots are especially impactful.

Edamame is another must-have kitchen staple. Not only good for guilt-free snacking, these young soybeans are rich in isoflavones, which help in reducing the chance of heart disease and diabetes – both conditions associated with chronic inflammation. If eating vegetables raw is not your thing, then try experimenting with vegetable juices, soups and colourful salads.

"TRY EXPERIMENTING WITH VEGETABLE JUICES, SOUPS AND COLOURFUL SALADS"

③ HERBS & SPICES

Although associated with bad breath, garlic is something you really need more of in your life. It is full of anti-inflammatory compounds and nutrients, and contains antioxidants that can neutralise the free radicals in the body. These are the molecules that steal electrons from other cells, thereby causing ageing and various diseases. Filled to the skin with sulphur compounds like diallyl disulphide, diallyl sulphide and allicin, all which have anti-inflammatory effects, this clever little bulb packs a punch like no other.

Hailed as the wonder spice, turmeric is a key ingredient to include in your cupboard. Bold in colour, it is powerful in its ability to reduce inflammation, particularly in relation to arthritis. This little super root contains the potent anti-inflammatory compound curcumin. This blocks the action of inflammatory molecules. Turmeric's antioxidants have also been linked to a reduction in the risk of glaucoma, cataracts and macular degeneration, and research has shown that people suffering with conditions like rheumatoid arthritis and inflammatory bowel disease can benefit massively from its healing effects. This warm, earthy spice is great for seasoning a variety of dishes and drinks as a powder or sliced up, but you can also purchase it in tablet form from health food shops.

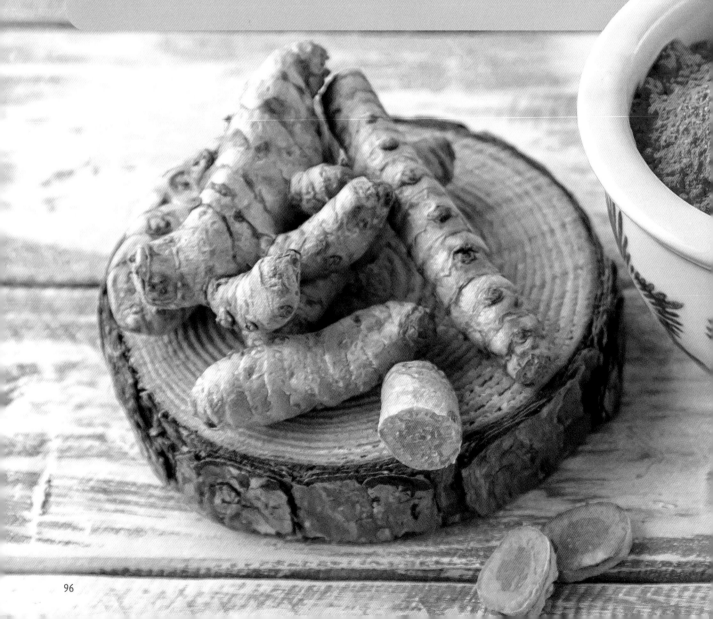

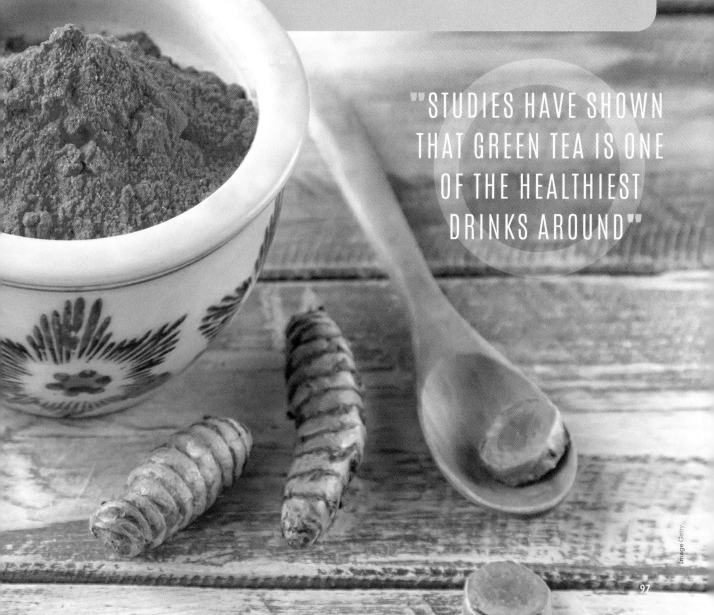

Another wonder root is ginger. Known for its anti-inflammatory abilities, it can aid in the reduction of swelling and is particularly useful for treating the symptoms of rheumatoid and osteoarthritis. Available in tablet form, ginger can also be ground up, sliced or grated, meaning it can be easily added to various dishes and beverages. Unfortunately, ginger biscuits have no anti-inflammatory benefits, although they do pair well with a cup of green tea!

Studies have shown that green tea is one of the healthiest drinks around. This is mainly due to the leaves' anti-inflammatory properties and high antioxidant count. It might be time to switch your English breakfast tea or latte for a cup of green tea, which is brimming with the unique plant compound epigallocatechin-3-gallate, known to hinder inflammation. This little leaf has also been linked to a reduced risk of heart disease, Alzheimer's, obesity and cancer.

In addition to these soothing options, you can also turn to cayenne, rosemary, honey or cinnamon to flavour your food and dampen inflammation at the same time.

"STUDIES HAVE SHOWN THAT GREEN TEA IS ONE OF THE HEALTHIEST DRINKS AROUND"

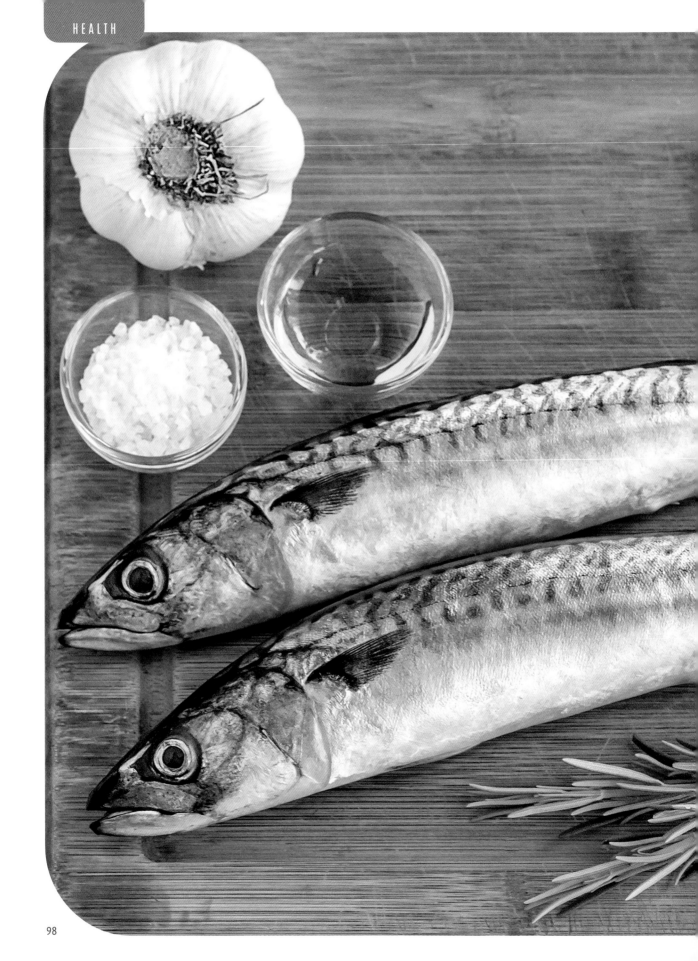

4 OILY FISH

Omega-3s are fantastic for lowering inflammation, and although they can be found in poultry like turkey or skinless chicken, they are most commonly associated with fish. All fish contain omega-3 fatty acids, but the leaders of the shoal are salmon, mackerel, anchovies, herring and sardines, all of which boast docosahexaenoic and eicosapentaenoic acid. These are long-chain omega-3 fatty acids that are metabolised by your body into compounds known as resolvins and protectins and have impressive anti-inflammatory properties. In addition fish is a fantastic source of protein and should be included in your diet at least three times a week for optimum health benefits.

What can get a little confusing is the relationship between omega-3s and omega-6 fatty acids. Omega-6 are the fatty acids your body needs for energy. We need to find these acids in what we eat as our body is unable to make them. They are responsible for aiding your body's growth and development and assisting in healing inflammation. Omega-6s are found in oils such as safflower, peanut, sunflower and corn. Omega-3s are the good fats found in fatty fish, flaxseeds and walnuts, among other things.

A healthy balance of the two omegas is vital; if you have too much omega-6 in your body and not enough omega-3, you risk creating an imbalance that can result in consistent inflammation caused by a pro-inflammatory response within the body.

Of the fatty fish, it is mackerel that is top of the school, boasting the highest content of omega-3 fatty acids with approximately 2.6 grams in every 100-gram serving. Wild salmon is another fishy favourite filled to the gills with omega-3s, and in the case of this pink swimmer, the omega-3 inside it is already in active form, meaning it will rapidly hone in on excess inflammation.

Although not an oily fish, oysters also contain essential omega-3 fatty acids and enjoying them as part of your diet can aid in prohibiting inflammatory cytokines in the body, soothe chronic inflammation and reduce your risk of serious disease.

Eating fish need not be a costly endeavour; tinned tuna is known to be one of the best anti-inflammatory foods with its high content of bioactive fatty acid and it is both simple and cheap to prepare. Just be sure that when it comes to dining on these water-loving wonders, the best way to keep your fatty acids well balanced is to always consume more omega-3 than omega-6, and if you are not a fan of eating fish, you can always purchase fish oil capsules from your health food shop or pharmacy.

> "TINNED TUNA IS KNOWN TO BE ONE OF THE BEST ANTI-INFLAMMATORY FOODS WITH ITS HIGH CONTENT OF BIOACTIVE FATTY ACID"

5 BEANS, LEGUMES & WHOLEGRAINS

Beans are a cost-effective, versatile and tasty way to add anti-inflammatory goodness to your meals. Not only can they be eaten hot or cold, in salads or soups or – every student's favourite – on toast, but they are also the perfect comfort food. Both the legume and bean families boast a high content of vitamins and minerals and are rich in fibre (foods high in fibre help to reduce the inflammatory hormone homocysteine). They are also packed with polyphenols, which work as antioxidants to combat inflammation.

Loaded with goodness, the options are many, including lentils, chickpeas, kidney beans, red beans, pinto beans, black-eyed peas and lentils. It is the black bean, however, that brings the most to the table. Studies have found that eating cooked black beans is linked to a greater diversity in gut bacteria, which in turn results in a decreased inflammatory response.

Like beans, quinoa, millet, amaranth and brown rice are also high in fibre, and on top of

"FIGURING OUT WHAT WORKS FOR YOUR INDIVIDUAL BODY IS IMPORTANT"

that they support the production of butyrate, a fatty acid that combats the genes related to insulin resistance and inflammation. Whole grains are also a great source of vitamin B, compensating for the loss of vitamins during the process of refinement.

Another magic bean is the cocoa bean, and as luck would have it studies have shown that dark chocolate (in moderation) could actually be good for you! Dark chocolate with a cocoa content of 70 per cent or more contains antioxidants, and chocolate's flavanols can assist in reducing inflammation and keeping the endothelial cells that line the arteries healthy. Better still, these antioxidants help boost your immunity by fighting inflammation and free radicals in the body, thus reducing the risk of several diseases. It is even said that chocolate can encourage healthier ageing (fingers crossed).

It is worth noting that some health food experts argue that legumes and beans can be responsible for causing inflammation. This is because they contain lectins that can be hard for the body to break down. However, by soaking, cooking and sprouting your beans first, you can actually neutralise the lectins inside them. Ultimately everybody is different, so figuring out what works for your individual body is important when choosing foods that will support your anti-inflammatory journey.

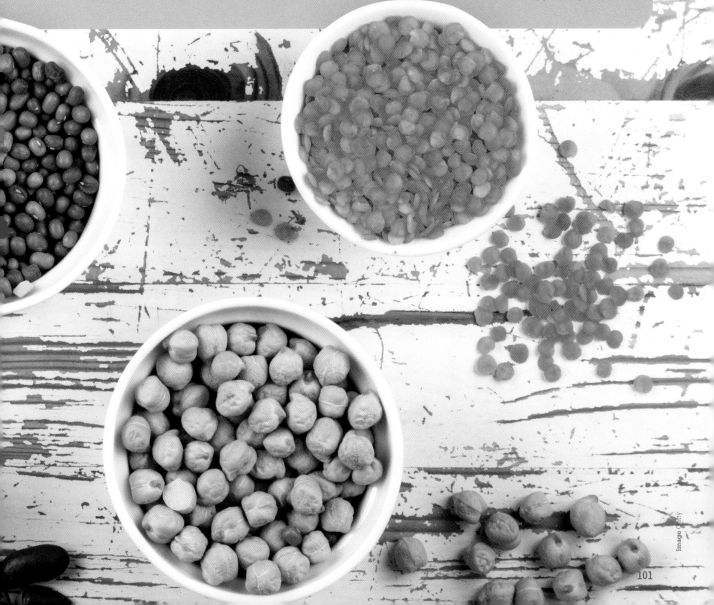

Image Getty

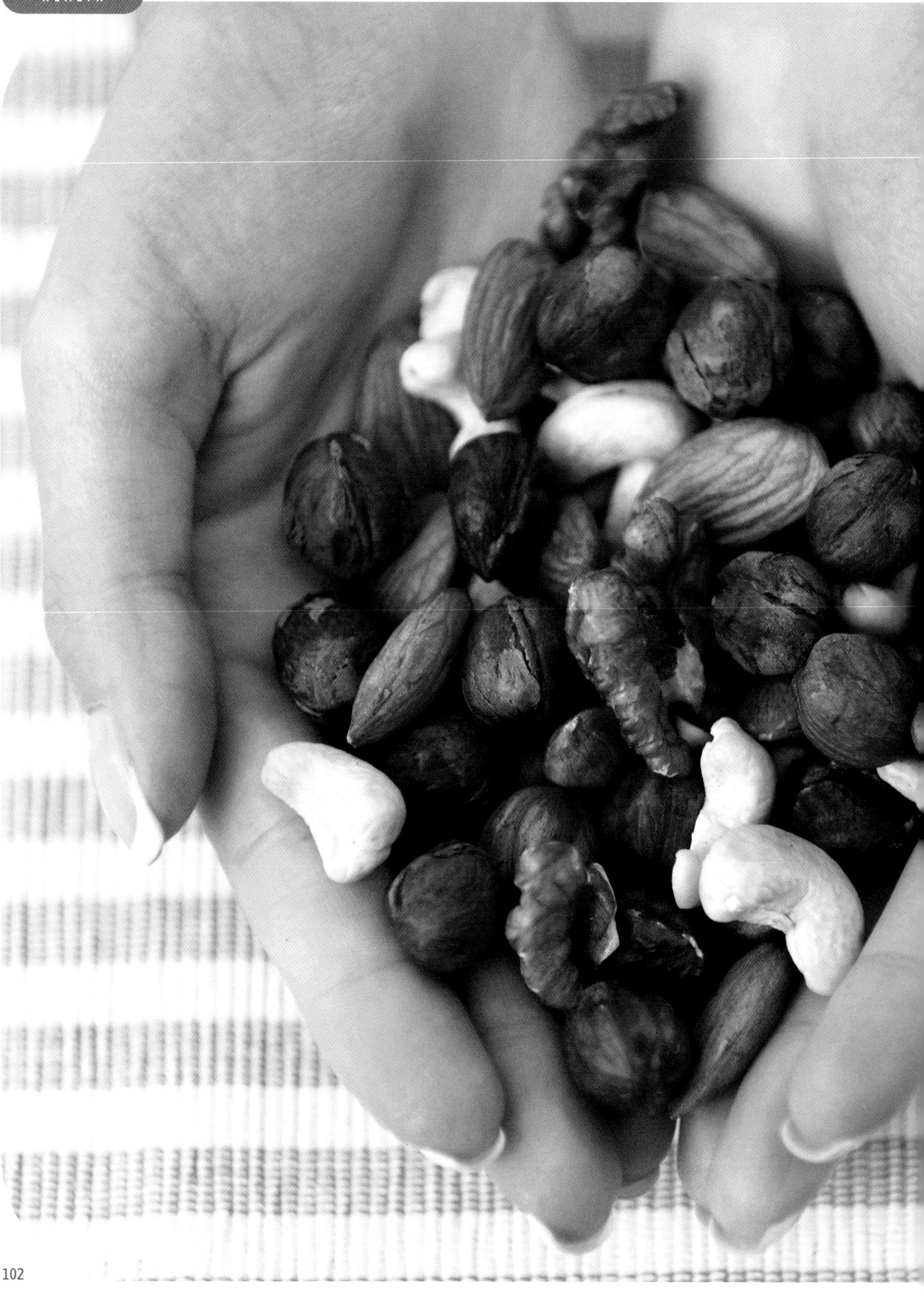

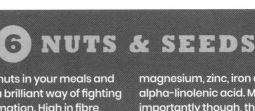

6 NUTS & SEEDS

Including nuts in your meals and snacks is a brilliant way of fighting off inflammation. High in fibre, magnesium, vitamin E, calcium, zinc and our old friend omega-3 fats, nuts offer numerous anti-inflammatory advantages. Hazelnuts, almonds, pistachios, walnuts and pecans are all filled with polyunsaturated and monounsaturated fats, ideal for reducing inflammation and in turn heart disease. Even peanuts can play a positive role in your diet – just take care to always buy raw nuts, as salted or roasted are unfortunately not as good for you, since they contain high levels of added salt and oil. It is the brain-shaped walnut, though, that really comes out of its shell with regards to reducing inflammation, due to its high content of alpha-linolenic acid. This is another variety of omega-3 fatty acid famed for its anti-inflammatory effects on the body.

Another anti-inflammatory powerhouse is the chia seed. These tiny little seeds come from the salvia hispanica plant and were favoured by the Maya and Aztec civilisations, namely for medicinal purposes but also as a food source. These fibre-rich seeds contain a health food shop's worth of vitamins and minerals including vitamins B1 and B3, phosphorus, calcium, magnesium, zinc, iron and alpha-linolenic acid. Most importantly though, they are packed with the antioxidants myricetin, chlorogenic acid, quercetin, kaempferol and caffeic acid. Together these antioxidants join together to combat the free radicals in the body. Not only do chia seeds aid in combating inflammation, they also assist in promoting positive bone health and weight management. They can be added to salads, yogurts, smoothies or porridge – or you can try using them to make a chia-seed pudding or add them to some overnight oats.

Known to help lower inflammation, flaxseed is a great source of both potassium and fibre. Full of essential fatty acids and lignans, this little seed contains approximately 6.3 grams of alpha-linolenic acid (ALA) in just one tablespoon. Its anti-inflammatory flavonoids can ease joint inflammation and arthritis, as well as skin conditions like psoriasis and eczema. Flaxseeds can be purchased whole, ground, as a capsule, in oil form or mixed in with other seeds. They can be added to smoothie bowls and yogurts, baked goods or as the secret ingredient to yummy vegan black-bean burgers for a double anti-inflammatory delicacy.

"FLAXSEED IS A GREAT SOURCE OF BOTH POTASSIUM AND FIBRE"

FOODS TO AVOID

What are the worst things we put in our bodies that may be contributing to problems with inflammation?

Our bodies are some of the most intricate systems known in nature. What we do, what we feel, and what we eat all play important roles in how our bodies function. Almost anything can impact how inflammation makes itself known. Perhaps the most simple method of dealing with inflammation that is causing us difficulty is to alter our diets.

There is no one diet which everyone can follow that will rid us of inflammation. In fact, because inflammation is so important to our health it would be foolish to try and get rid of it entirely. But there are some simple changes that we can all make to ensure that our immune system works for us and not against us. Diet can be the most effective method at our disposal.

The first change to make is to be mindful of what you consume. It is easy to graze throughout the day and never notice exactly what it is you are eating. By focusing on each thing you eat, you might pick up on specific relationships between how you feel and a single food type. Some people suffer from diffuse food allergy symptoms that make them feel dizzy, nauseous, and itchy after exposure to a particular food. If you often suffer an upset stomach after eating the same ingredient, then it may be causing an inflammatory response in your gut. Avoiding it in the future will improve your health.

Sometimes, we will find a range of food that does not agree with us and this is often down to an immune response causing inflammation. Histamine is a natural product of your body and plays many roles in our biology. It is best known for its role in causing the symptoms of allergies. For some people, foods that are rich in histamines will cause inflammation. Avoid foods that are high in histamines like smoked meats, aged cheese, dried fruits, avocados, and spinach. Alcohols and fermented foods also have histamines, and alcohol blocks the enzyme that naturally removes histamines from the body.

Research has intensified in recent years on the relationship between food and inflammation. As well as the specific foods that we know may trigger inflammation in an individual, some groups of food are being identified that may be best for you to limit or avoid in your diet. Diet will not cure everything and must be considered as part of an active and happy life, but there are some changes you could make to improve inflammation.

Achieving a healthy weight can be hard for some but it is important to bear in mind that obesity has a large role to play in inflammation. Some researchers consider obesity itself to be a source of low level chronic inflammation. By reducing the level of fatty tissue in our bodies to a healthy level, we remove

Sometimes it is the food we crave the most which can have the worst impacts on our health and cause inflammation

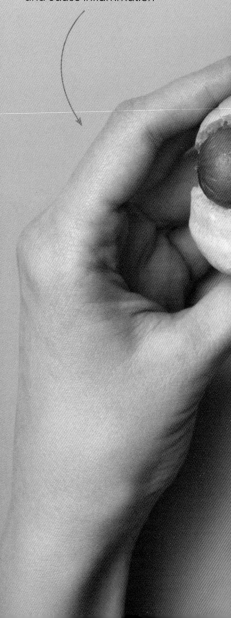

this source of inflammation. Diet is key to reaching a weight that supports our health and reduces chronic inflammation.

Sugar

///////

One of the best ways to change our diet to improve health is to reduce the level of sugar consumed throughout the day. Humans have sweet teeth and in recent decades, the food we buy has become increasingly sweet with more sugar being added during production. Snacks that include lots of sugar taste good but do not satisfy our hunger for long, and this can lead to eating even more of them.

This is bad for inflammation as many studies have shown that excess sugar in our blood triggers the immune response. High sugar diets have been linked to rheumatoid arthritis, multiple sclerosis, inflammatory bowel disease, and low-grade chronic inflammation. Increased levels of sugar induce the body to release chemicals linked to the immune response and inflammation is linked to all of these conditions, and more. It is not possible, or desirable, to cut all sugar from our diet. There are ways to avoid it becoming too much, however.

A can of a sugary soft drink can contain nine teaspoons of sugar – the entire recommended daily amount for a man. Other obvious foods to avoid are sweets and candies that contain a lot of sugar and few other nutrients. Cakes and pastries often contain far more sugar than you might expect. Cutting these out can be difficult, but if you need a sweet treat, try fresh fruit as an alternative.

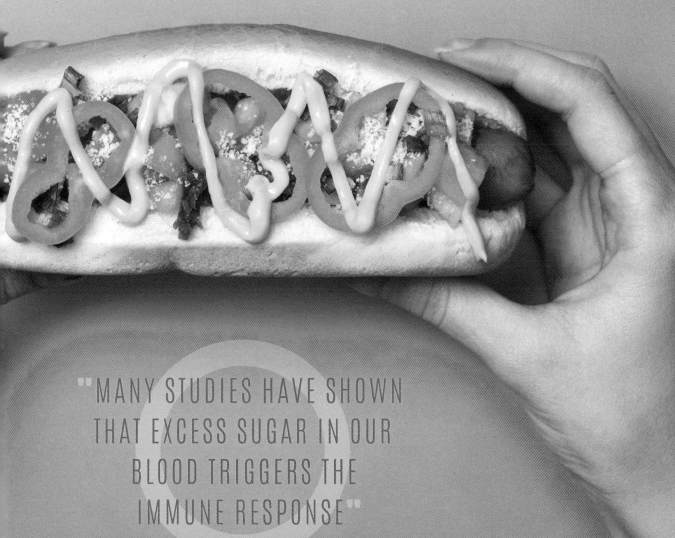

"MANY STUDIES HAVE SHOWN THAT EXCESS SUGAR IN OUR BLOOD TRIGGERS THE IMMUNE RESPONSE"

Foods that are high in antioxidants are recommended to lower inflammation. Sometimes you will see chocolate included on this list. Be careful however – many chocolates are high in sugar. Very dark chocolate in small amounts may be beneficial, but not a large amount of very sweet milk or white chocolate.

Another source of sugars is from simple and overly refined carbohydrates. These are easily broken down in the body into sugars and cause sharp increases in blood glucose levels, which are associated with inflammation. Refined carbohydrates are found in things like white flour and many pastas. Try to replace these with wholemeal alternatives as these contain complex carbohydrates that take longer to be metabolised and do not raise your blood glucose so much.

Fats

Fats have been heavily vilified in the discussion of diets. They are high calorie and were blamed for a long time as the main cause

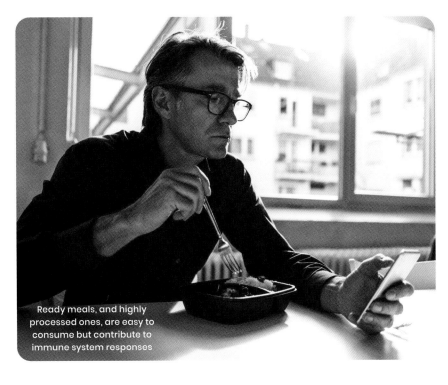

Ready meals, and highly processed ones, are easy to consume but contribute to immune system responses

of obesity. Fats are, however vital, for the functioning of the human body. Which fats we consume and in what quantities is more important than simply cutting out all fat from our diet.

It is known that some fatty acids cause inflammation by helping bacterial toxins cross from the flora in our gut into the bloodstream. The immune system detects this and causes a short-term inflammatory

response. Others mimic the chemicals which mediate the immune system and trigger a response. Long-chain fatty acids are thought to cause stress on our cells that prompts the immune system to activate.

Working out which fats you should eat may seem difficult at first. An easy way to regulate your fat intake is to avoid fried foods. These have high levels of saturated and trans fats which can cause inflammation, and may change the microbiome of your gut in a way that further increases inflammation. Look out for saturated and trans fats in the nutrition information on your food.

Foods which have 'hydrogenated' fats listed in the ingredients have high levels of trans fats in them. Some margarines contain these, as well as some snack foods. Try to replace margarine and butter with an olive oil spread.

Animal fats, which are unsaturated, are found in red meat and can also contribute to inflammation. Conversely, the omega-3 fatty acids found in many oily fish reduce the immune response. The oils we choose to

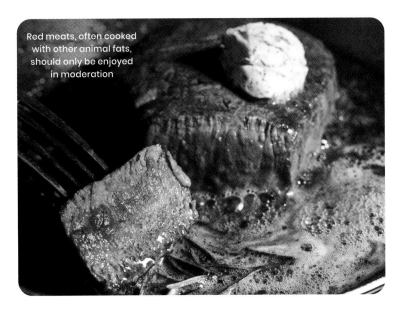

Red meats, often cooked with other animal fats, should only be enjoyed in moderation

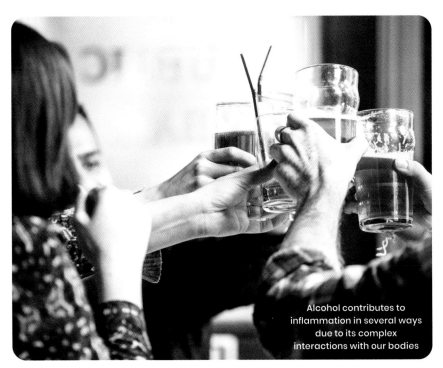

Alcohol contributes to inflammation in several ways due to its complex interactions with our bodies

Snack foods are also often a mix of all the ingredients we should avoid to reduce inflammation, but because they are designed to tempt us it is easy to overeat. When you want a snack, try to make one for yourself – it will likely satisfy you longer than a bag of crisps or cake bar.

Research

The role of food in inflammation is still an area of active research. It was only recently that the importance of the bacteria in our gut for our health was established. More work is constantly being done, so it is important to keep up to date on what the science is telling us about the relationship of diet to inflammation. It is best to read reputable journals and science websites for the most up-to-date information available. At first the amount of advice may seem formidable but remember, you do not have to make every change to your diet at once. Everyone is individual in their needs. No one diet will work for everyone. Make a few small changes and see which ones work for you.

cook with also contribute to fat-caused inflammation. Avoid cooking oils with too much omega-6 in them, like corn and soya bean oil. Extra-virgin olive oil has a lower proportion of omega-6 fatty acids.

Processed foods

We are living increasingly busy lives and it is all too easy to fall into the habit of buying food that is ready made. They may be convenient but processed foods may lead to inflammation, because they contain multiple chemicals which can provoke the immune system into action. These are often added during production to improve the taste and shelf-life of highly-processed foods. Eating too many high- or ultra-processed foods changes the makeup of the bacteria we require in our digestive system and this impacts our immune system for the worse.

The simplest way to avoid highly-processed foods is to make as much as you can for yourself. Try to use fresh ingredients as the basis of most of your meals. Avoid foods that no longer look like they were ever ingredients to begin with. Look for a short list of ingredients on the back of any meals you do buy and pay particular attention to the levels of salt, fats, and sugar.

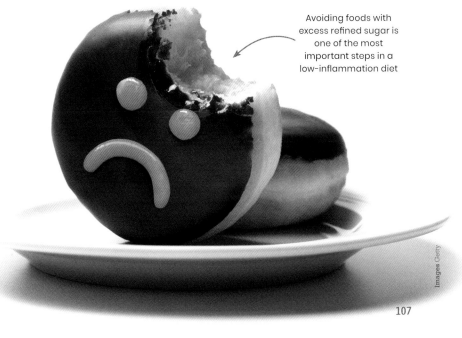

Avoiding foods with excess refined sugar is one of the most important steps in a low-inflammation diet

Images Getty

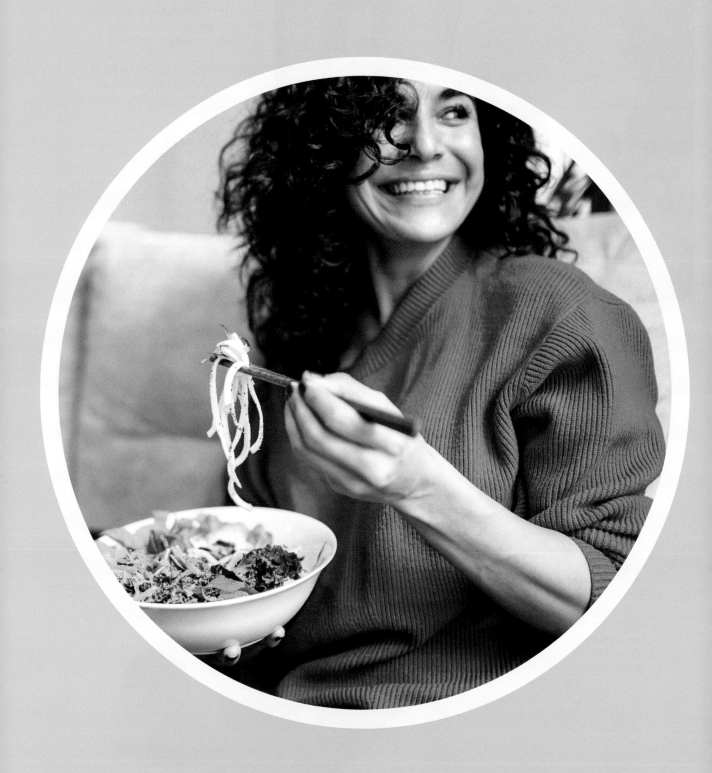

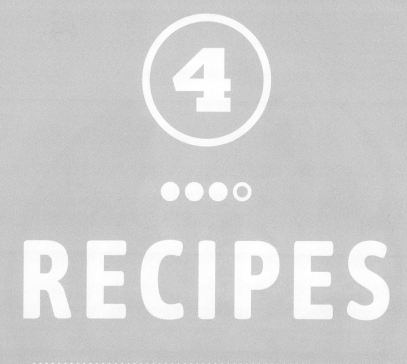

4

●●●●○

RECIPES

//

*Embrace anti-inflammatory eating habits
with this selection of delicious recipes!
Featuring meat-free, vegan, dairy-free
and gluten-free options.*

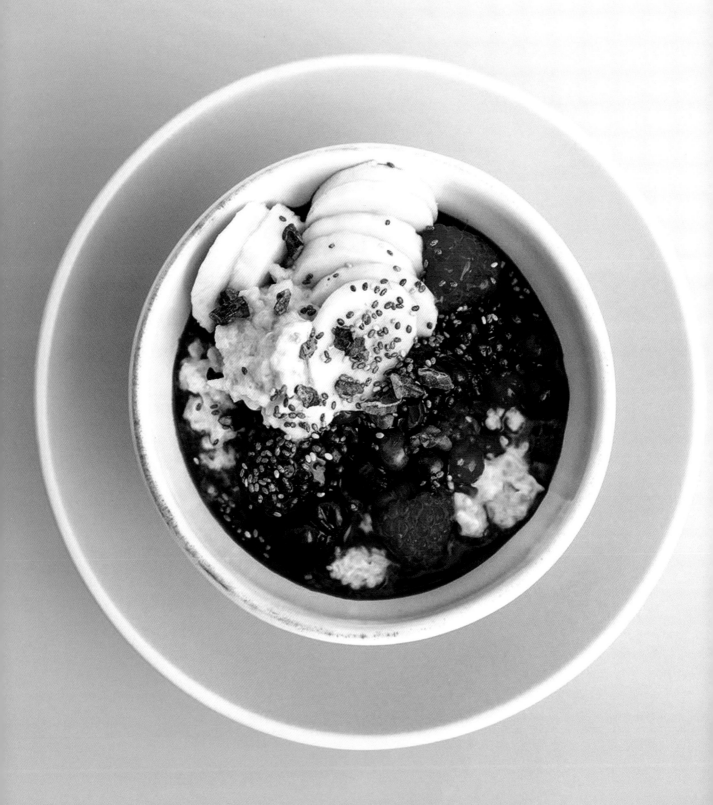

SUPER BERRY BREAKFAST BOWL

The chia seeds and walnut add a lovely textural contrast to the oats and compote

SERVES 1 - READY IN 25 MINS

DF GF VE

Ingredients

- **80 g** | **½ cups** | **2.8 oz** frozen berries
- **Zest** ½ orange and a squeeze of juice
- **50 g** | **½ cups** | **1.7 oz** gluten free oats
- **100 ml** | **½ cups** | **3.5 oz** coconut yogurt (dairy free)
- ¼ banana, sliced
- **½ tsp** chia seeds
- **½ tsp** cacao nibs
- **2 tbsp** walnuts, chopped
- **Handful of** berries to garnish

Method

1. Put the berries, orange zest and juice into a small pan and cook on a medium heat for 5 minutes until softened.

2. Stir the oats into the yogurt and leave to sit for 15 minutes. Top with the warm compote and garnish with banana, extra berries, chia seeds, cocoa nibs and walnuts.

PROTEIN POWER

According to the British Nutrition Foundation the average adult needs about 0.6 g of protein per kilo of bodyweight a day, which is equal to about 56 g of protein a day for men and 45 g for women. The rest of the protein we eat is used to give us energy. For vegans, only 10% of their calories need to come from proteins. These come from legumes, whole grains, nuts and seeds. Just 100 g of chickpeas provides you with 18% of the daily value of protein. Some of the best sources of protein include quinoa, meat alternatives such as tofu, pulses such as lentils, hemp seeds, buckwheat, oats and brown rice. Many people think you can't get enough protein on a plant-based diet, but they could not be more wrong. Even if you're active you can get more than enough protein – even professional athletes are converting to vegan diets.

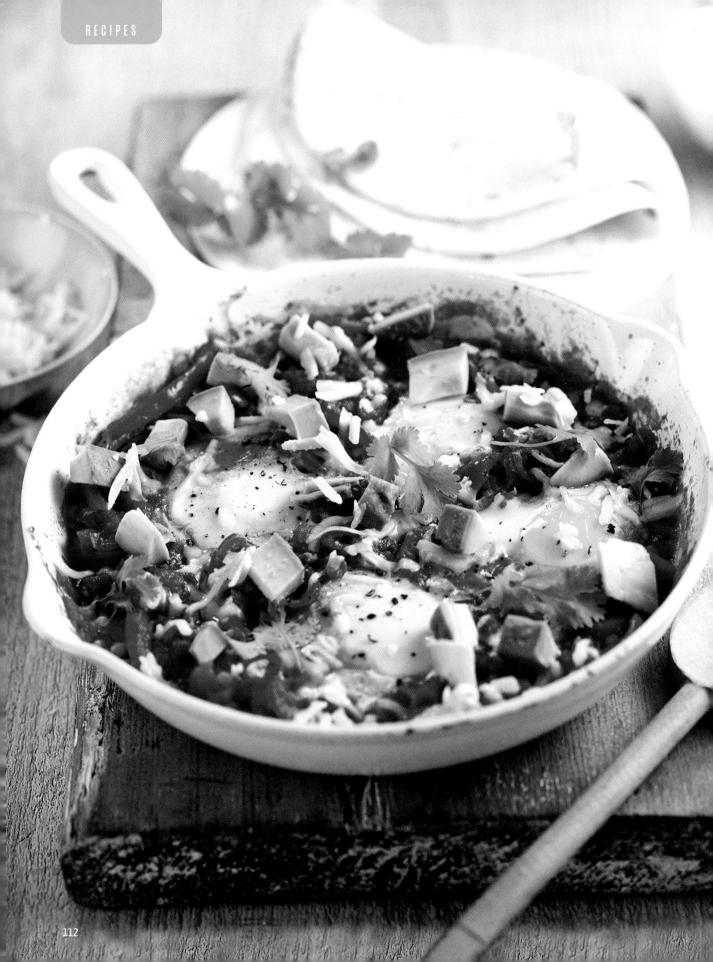

HUEVOS RANCHEROS

An easy Mexican style breakfast that will keep you going until lunch

SERVES 4 - READY IN 30 MINS

GF

Ingredients

- **400 g | 14.1 oz** chopped tomatoes
- **100 g | 3.5 oz** vegetarian cheese, grated
- **1** onion, finely chopped
- **1** garlic clove, diced
- **1** red pepper, thinly sliced
- **1** red chilli, thinly sliced
- **4** eggs
- **4** gluten free flour tortillas
- **1** avocado, sliced
- **Handful of** coriander leaves to serve

Method

1. Heat the oil in a frying pan over a medium heat and add the onion, garlic, red pepper and chilli with a pinch of salt. Cook for 5 min until beginning to soften then pour over the tomatoes and cook for a further 5 min.

2. Make 4 holes in the tomato mixture and crack the eggs into them. Cover with a lid and cook for 5min until the eggs are set.

3. To serve, heat each flour tortilla in a separate pan for 1 min until slightly crisp. Place on a plate and spoon over one of the eggs with some tomato. Top with the avocado, cheese and coriander and season.

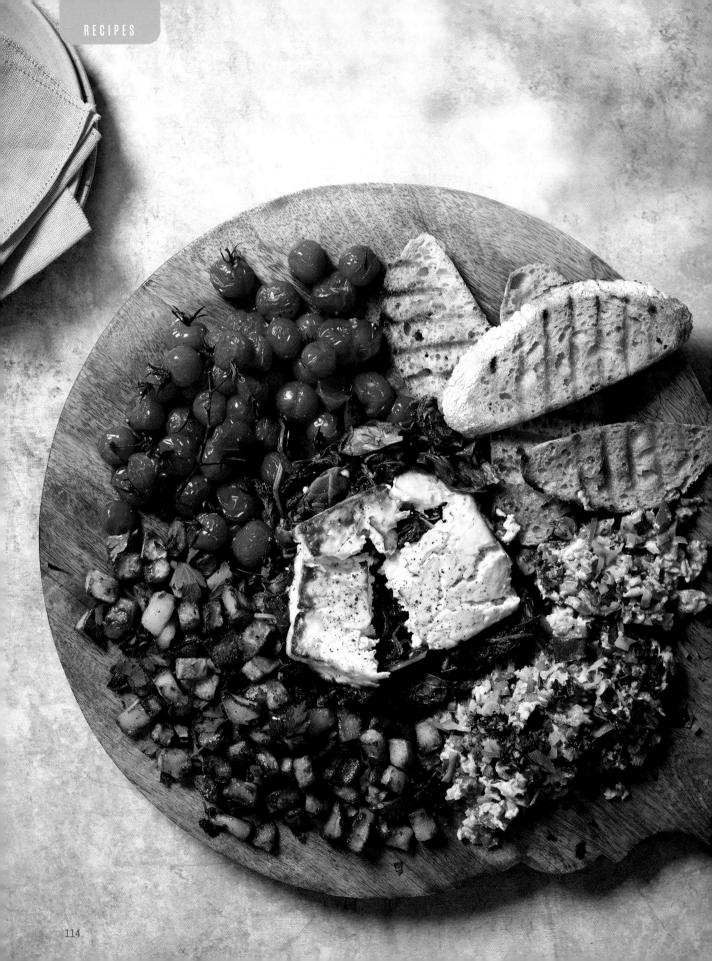

VEGGIE BRUNCH BOARD

Host a brunch and serve the best bits of a veggie fry-up

SERVES 4 - READY IN 55 MINS

Ingredients

- **2** baking potatoes, peeled & cubed
- **400 g** | **14.1 oz** cherry tomatoes
- **200 g** | **7 oz** feta
- **2 tbsp** olive oil, plus extra, to drizzle
- **260 g** | **9.2 oz** spinach
- **1** garlic clove
- Toast, to serve

For the Spiced Scrambled Eggs

- **Knob** of butter
- **1** green pepper, finely chopped
- **2** spring onions, finely chopped
- **1** large tomato, deseeded and finely chopped
- **4** eggs, lightly beaten
- **1 tbsp** flat-leaf parsley, finely chopped
- **Pinch** of mild chilli flakes

Method

1. Heat the oven to 180°C/350°F/Gas Mark 4, leaving a large cast-iron pan in it while it comes to temperature. Toss the potatoes in half the oil and season liberally. Add to the cast-iron pan, return to the oven and cook for 30 mins, turning after 15 mins.

2. Season and mix the cherry tomatoes with the remaining oil. Roast for 15 mins.

3. Drizzle the feta with a little oil, wrap it in foil and bake for 15 mins. Remove the potatoes and tomatoes and keep warm. Heat the grill to maximum, uncover the feta and grill for 10 mins, until golden.

4. Steam the spinach for 2 mins, until wilted. Stir through the garlic.

5. For the eggs, melt the butter in a pan big enough to take all the ingredients and gently fry the pepper and spring onions for 2 mins, stirring. Add the chopped tomato and cook gently for 5 mins. Pour in the eggs. Stir gently and, as they start to scramble, add the parsley and chilli. Assemble everything on a sharing board and let everyone help themselves.

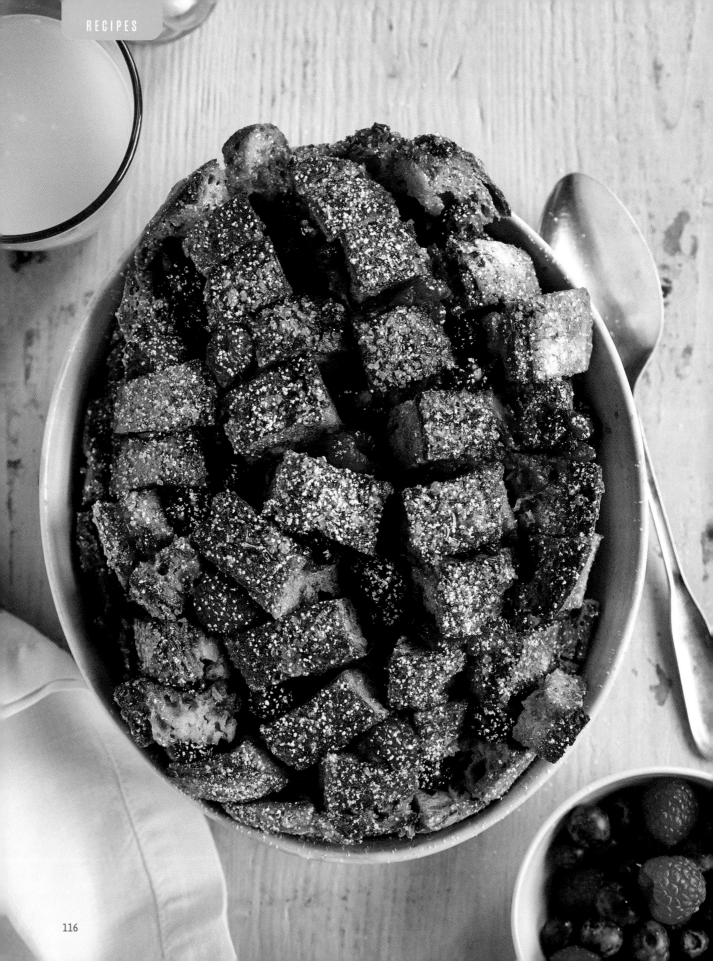

FRENCH TOAST BERRY LOAF

Packed with fruits, our French toast berry loaf might become your new go-to tear-and-share recipe

SERVES **6** - READY IN **1** HOUR PLUS SOAKING

Ingredients

- **500 g** | **17 oz** sourdough loaf
- **2** large eggs, plus **1** egg yolk (save the white for glazing)
- **100 ml** | **¼ cup + 2 tbsp** | **3.5 oz** double cream
- **250 ml** | **1 cup + 1 tbsp** | **8.8 oz** whole milk
- **1 tbsp** vanilla bean paste
- **1 tsp** cinnamon
- **1 tbsp** vanilla bean paste
- **150 ml** | **5.3 oz** blueberries
- **100 ml** | **3.5 oz** raspberries
- **1 tbsp** demerara sugar
- **1 tbsp** tbsp maple syrup, plus more to serve
- **1** icing sugar, to dust

Method

1. Heat the oven to 180°C / 350°F / Gas Mark 4. Make deep slices across the loaf in both directions, ensuring you don't go all the way through, to create a grid pattern.

2. Mix the eggs and egg yolk, cream, milk, vanilla and cinnamon in a jug. Place the bread in an ovenproof dish and pour the egg mix over. Leave this to soak for at least 20 mins or ideally overnight, to enhance the flavours.

3. Scatter half the fruit into the bread, pushing it into the grooves. Spoon over any remaining liquid that hasn't been absorbed. Brush with egg white, sprinkle over the demerara sugar and bake for 45-50 mins, until crunchy and set.

4. Scatter over the remaining fruit, drizzle over the maple syrup and dust with icing sugar. Serve warm on serving plates with more syrup, if liked.

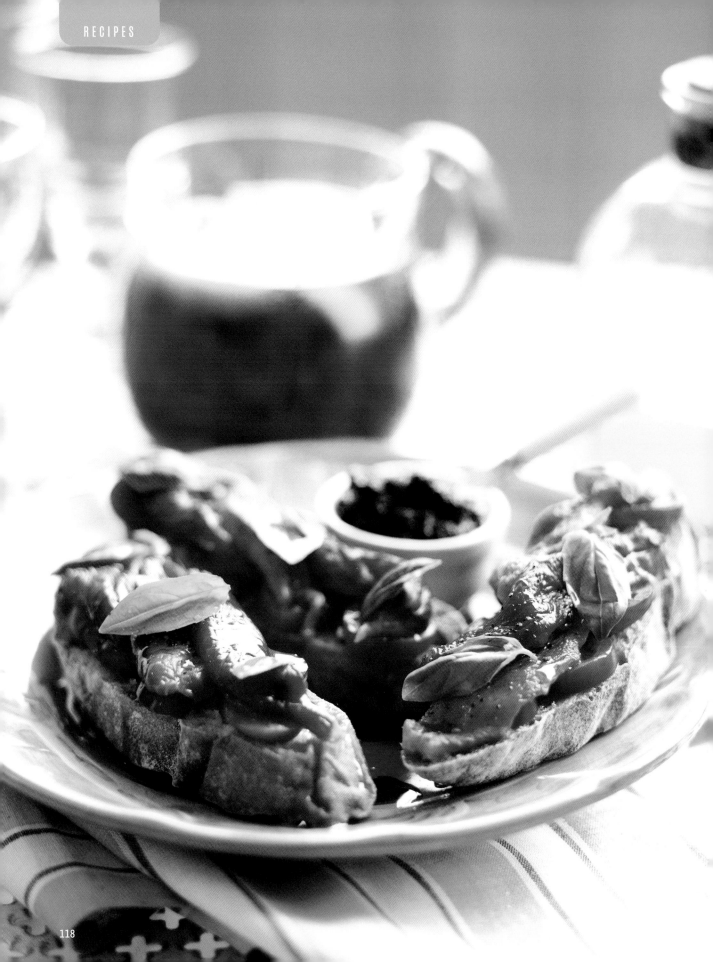

ROASTED PEPPER &
GARLIC BRUSCHETTA

While it takes a little time to roast the peppers and garlic, the wait is worth it for this wonderful mix of fresh flavours

SERVES **8** - READY IN **55** MINS

DF VE

Ingredients

- **1** bulb of garlic
- **3** red or yellow peppers
- **8** slices ciabatta, toasted
- **16** cherry tomatoes, sliced
- Basil leaves
- Olive oil, to drizzle
- Black olive tapenade, to serve

Method

1. Heat the oven to 200°C / 400°F / Gas Mark 6. Wrap the garlic in foil and put in a roasting tin with the peppers. Cook for 40 mins, until the peppers are soft and slightly blackened.

2. Put the peppers in a bowl, cover with clingfilm and leave to steam for 10 mins.

3. Once cool enough to handle, peel away the skins from the peppers, and the tops and seeds. Cut into strips and set aside.

4. Remove the garlic from the foil and squeeze the cloves out from their skins. Spread one onto each slice of ciabatta, then put tomato slices on top, followed by strips of pepper, basil leaves, seasoning and a drizzle of olive oil. Serve with the tapenade on the side to dip into.

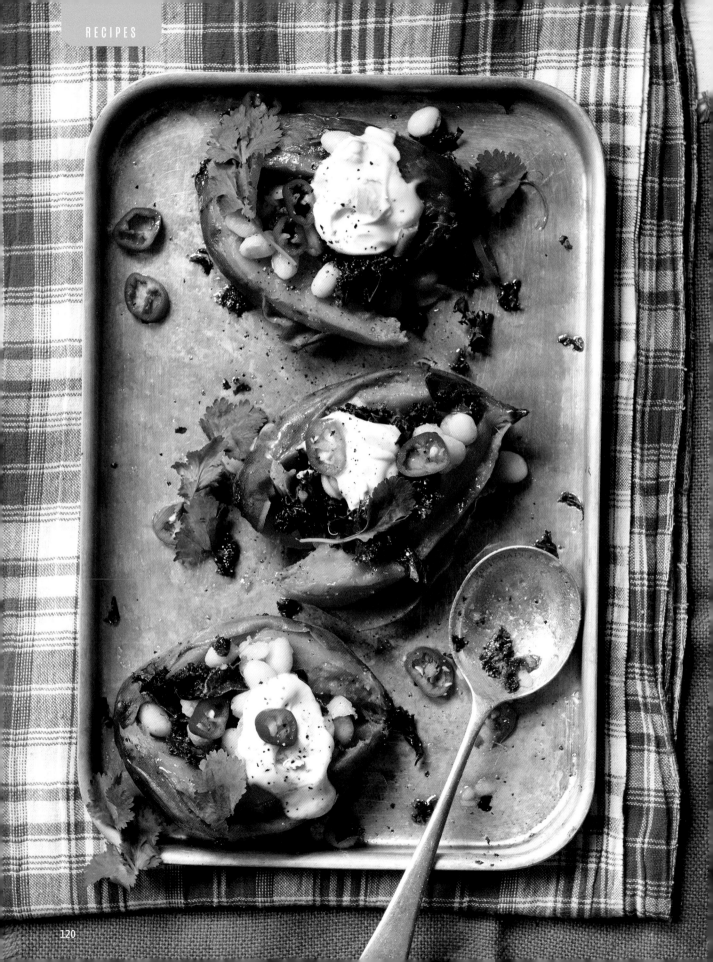

BAKED & STUFFED SWEET POTATOES

These healthy baked potatoes are loaded with greens and crème fraîche for a fresh and zesty twist

SERVES 4 - READY IN 1 HOUR

GF

Ingredients

- **4** sweet potatoes, cleaned
- **60 g** | **¼ cup** | **2 oz** butter, cut into 4 chunks
- **4 tbsp** maple syrup
- **100 g** | **3.5 oz** kale
- **400 ml** | **14 oz** can white beans, drained
- **2 tbsp** olive oil
- **120 ml** | **½ cup** | **4.2 oz** crème fraîche
- **1** bunch of coriander, stalks removed
- **1** red chilli, sliced

Method

1. Heat the oven to 180°C / 350°F / Gas Mark 4. Tear 4 sheets of foil big enough to cover sweet potatoes. Place the potatoes in centre of the foil and cut lengthways down the centre. Top with the butter, drizzle over the maple syrup and sprinkle over salt and pepper. Cook for 40-45 mins until soft.

2. Just before the sweet potatoes are ready, put the kale and beans on a baking tray and drizzle over the olive oil. Bake for 10-15 mins until cooked through.

3. Serve each of the potato parcels, opened, with the kale and beans, and a good dollop of crème fraîche on top. Scatter over the coriander and sliced red chilli.

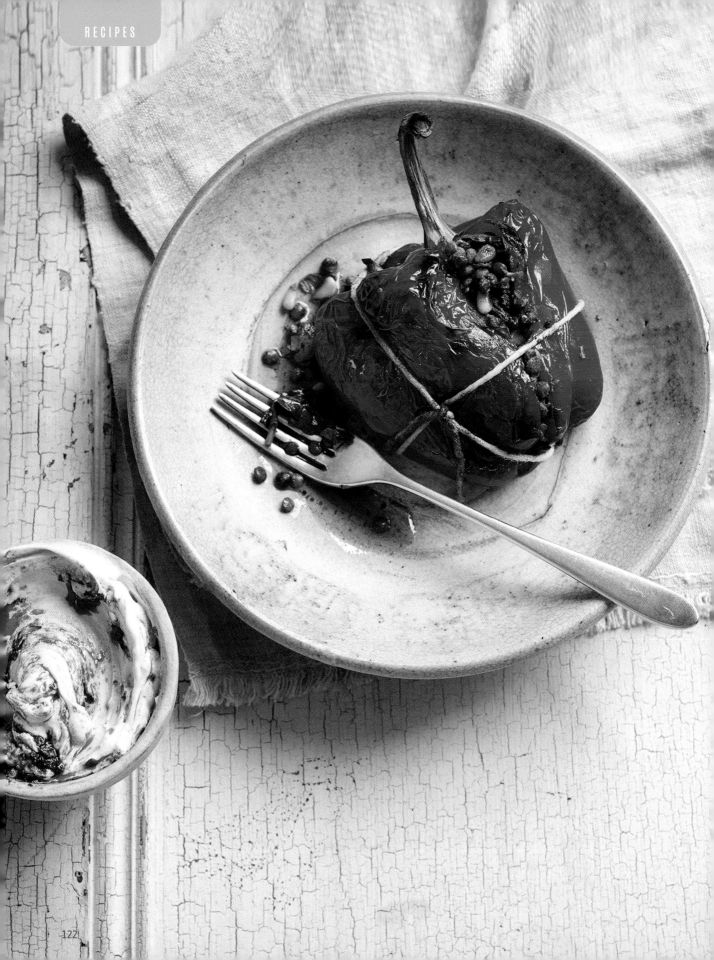

STUFFED PEPPERS
WITH HARISSA YOGURT

This aromatic yogurt will become your new favourite side

SERVES 6 - READY IN 1 HOUR   GF

Ingredients

For the Peppers

- **1** onion, chopped
- **1 tbsp** olive oil
- **2** cloves garlic, finely chopped
- **½ tsp** ground cinnamon
- **½ tsp** ground cumin
- **200 g** | **7 oz** puy lentils, rinsed
- **400 ml** | **1 ½ cups + 3 tbsp** | **13.5 oz** gluten free vegetable stock
- **150 g** | **5.3 oz** spinach leaves
- **2 tbsp** raisins
- **2 tbsp** pine nuts, toasted in a dry pan
- **2 tbsp** chopped mint
- **2 tbsp** chopped parsley
- **6** red peppers, halved and deseeded

For the Yogurt

- **2 tbsp** harissa paste
- **300 g** | **1 cup + 3 tbsp** | **10.6 oz** Greek yogurt

Method

1. Heat the oven to 200°C / 400°F / Gas Mark 6. Gently soften the onion in the oil for 10 mins. Add the garlic, cinnamon and cumin and cook for 1 min. Stir in the lentils and stock. Bring to the boil, then simmer for 15 mins until the lentils are tender, but still hold their shape.

2. Fold in the spinach just before removing from the heat, letting it wilt. Stir in the raisins, pine nuts, mint and parsley, and season to taste.

3. Lay the peppers out, cut sides up, and fill with the lentil mixture. Pair up the halves and tie together with string. For extra security, wrap the peppers tightly in oiled foil. Place in a roasting tin, in the oven, for about 30 mins. Swirl the harissa into the yogurt and serve with the peppers.

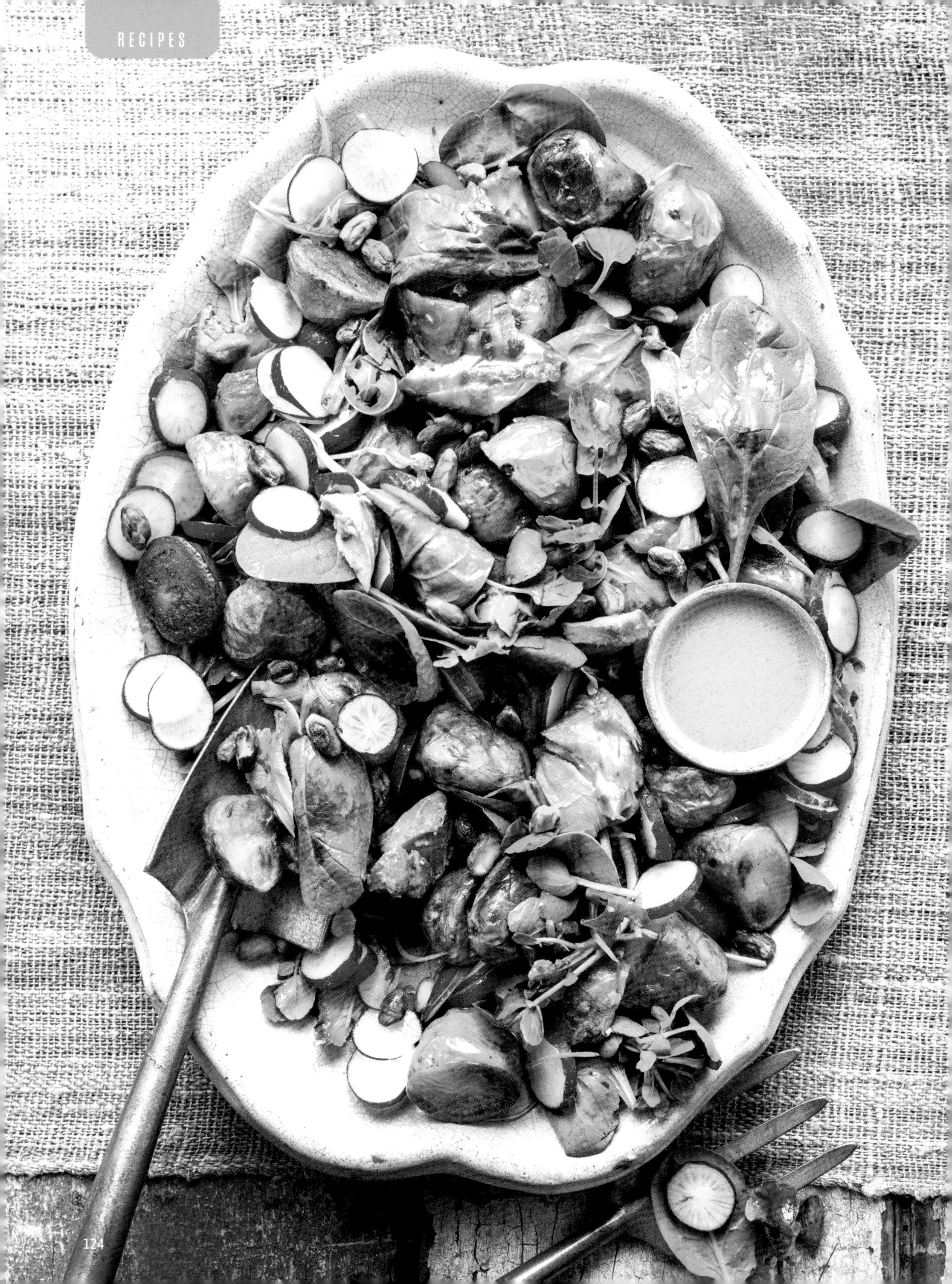

HOT-SMOKED SALMON & POTATO SALAD

Any leftovers of this light, bright salad would make a tasty packed lunch to take to work the next day

SERVES 4 - READY IN 45 MINS

DF GF

Ingredients

- **500 g** | **17 oz** baby new potatoes, halved
- **1** garlic clove, crushed
- **2 tbsp** olive oil
- **100 g** | **3.5 oz** pistachios
- **¼ tbsp** sea salt
- **200 g** | **7 oz** French beans (optional)
- **125 g** | **4.4 oz** watercress, rocket and spinach
- **200 g** | **7 oz** hot-smoked salmon, flaked
- **200 g** | **7 oz** radishes, trimmed and sliced

For the Dressing

- **2 tbsp** virgin olive oil
- **2 tbsp** white wine vinegar
- **2 tbsp** maple syrup
- **2 tbsp** Dijon mustard

Method

1. Heat the oven to 220°C / 420°F / Gas Mark 7. Roast the potatoes with the garlic and oil for 30 mins, until they're tender and golden.

2. Spread the pistachios onto a baking tray, and scatter with the sea salt and 3tbsp water. Cook in the oven for 3-5 mins, until the nuts are toasted and the water has evaporated. Microwave the French beans, if using, with 2tbsp water for 3 mins, until tender; drain.

3. Arrange the watercress, rocket and spinach on a platter. Top with the potatoes, pistachios, French beans, flaked salmon and radishes. Put the dressing ingredients in a jar with 2tbsp water and season. Seal and shake to mix.

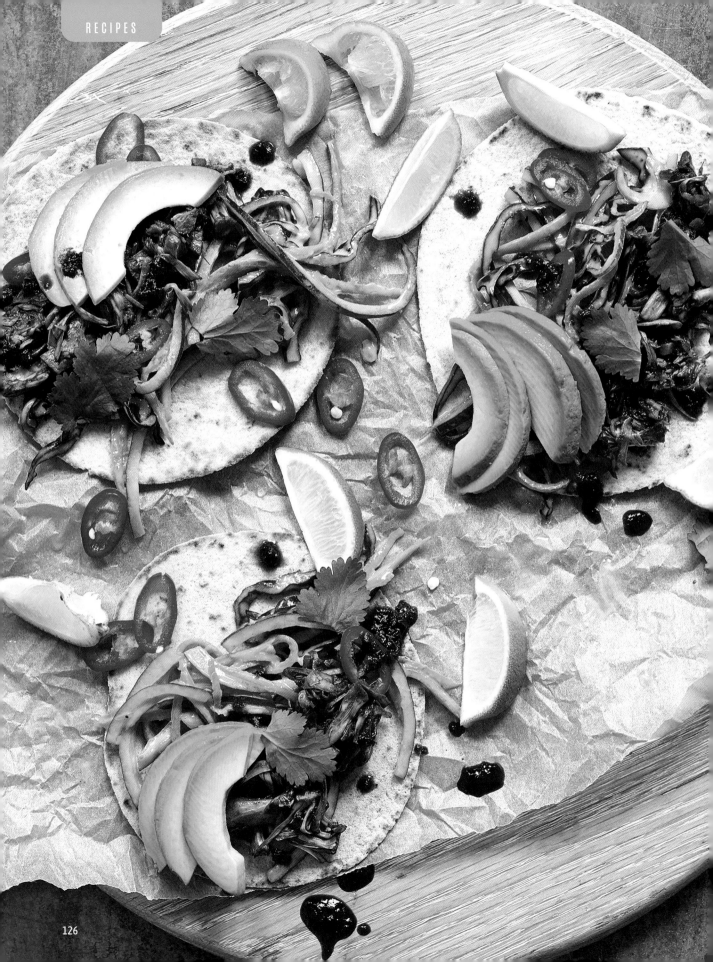

JACKFRUIT TACOS

You won't miss pulled pork with these juicy jackfruit tacos

SERVES 4 - READY IN 20 MINS

DF VE

Ingredients

- **800 g** | **5 cups** | **28 oz** tinned jackfruit
- **200 ml** | **¾ cups** | **7 fl oz** barbecue sauce
- ½ red cabbage, shredded
- **2** carrots, julienned
- **1** red onion, finely sliced
- **2 tbsp** egg-free mayonnaise
- **1 tsp** Dijon mustard
- Juice of **1** lime
- **12** soft corn tacos
- **1** avocado, sliced
- **1** red chilli, sliced
- Coriander leaves
- Lime wedges

Method

1. Drain and rinse the jackfruit, then use two forks to shred the fruit to resemble pulled pork. Put the jackfruit and most of the barbecue sauce in a small pan over a medium heat to warm through. Stir often to ensure the jackfruit is well coated in the sauce. Once hot, set aside and keep warm until needed.

2. To make a crunchy slaw, toss the veg through the mayo, mustard and lime juice. Season well.

3. Toast the tacos for 1 minute on either side in a frying pan. Then, spoon some slaw into the centre of each, and top with a good helping of jackfruit. Serve the warm tacos with the sliced avocado, fresh chilli, coriander leaves, the remaining barbecue sauce, and a couple of lime wedges on the side.

MYTH: NOT ENOUGH PROTEIN IN PLANTS

One of the most common myths about changing to a plant-based or vegan diet is that if you're not eating meat, fish and eggs, you won't have enough protein in your diet, but this is not true. In fact, plants produce 10 times more protein per acre than meat. You can get the same amount of protein in half a cup of beans as you can by eating an ounce of meat. The main difference between proteins like meat, fish and eggs and plant-based proteins in vegetables, whole grains, legumes, nuts and seeds is that the former are complete proteins (they contain all nine amino acids), whereas the latter are incomplete proteins. However, this does not mean you need them in your diet. Plant-based foods have enough protein in them. You just need to ensure your diet is varied so that you're getting enough. These proteins are incomplete because they can't build new proteins in your body by themselves, but combine a plant-based protein like peanut butter with wholemeal bread and voila! You have a complete protein.

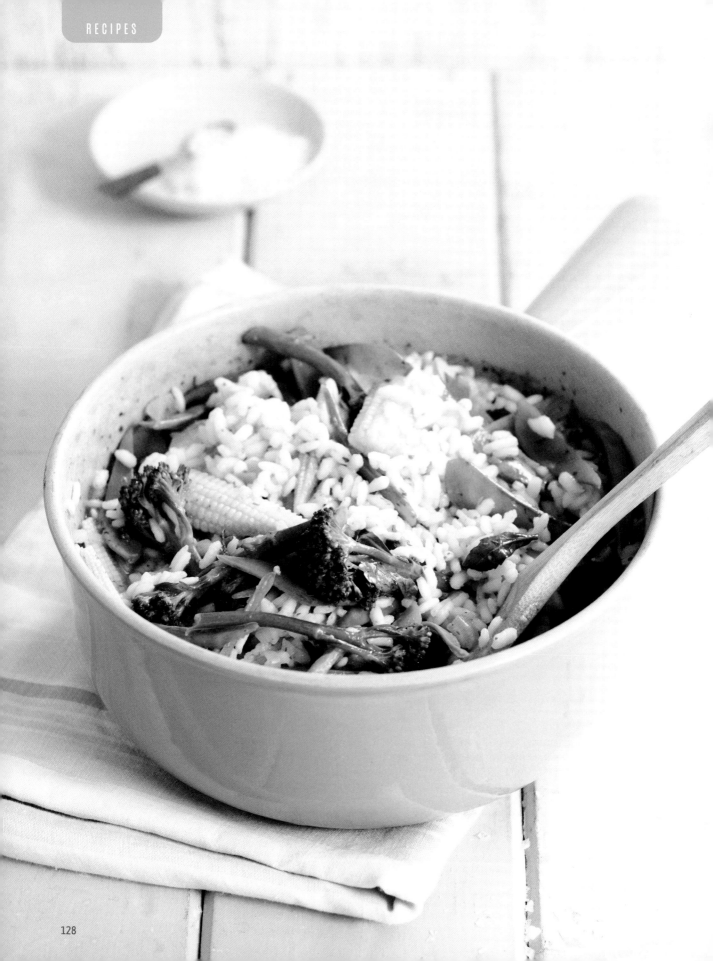

LEMON &
BROCCOLI RISOTTO

Why not add a splash of vegan white wine?

SERVES 4 - READY IN 30 MINS

DF VE

Ingredients

- **3 tbsp** rapeseed oil
- **1** small onion, finely diced
- **1** garlic clove, crushed
- **300 g** | **1 ½ cups** | **10 oz** risotto rice
- **1.2 litres** vegetable stock
- **200 g** | **2 cups** | **7 oz** tenderstem broccoli
- **100 g** | **¾ cups** | **3.5 oz** baby sweetcorn
- **100 g** | **1 cups** | **3.5 oz** mangetout
- Zest and juice ½ unwaxed lemon

Method

1. Heat the oil in a frying pan, add the onion and cook over a low heat for 5 minutes until the onion is soft. Add the garlic and cook for a few seconds, then stir in the rice.

2. Heat the stock in another pan and bring to simmering point. Add the stock to the rice, one ladleful at a time, stirring continuously until it has been absorbed and the rice is creamy. When almost all the stock has been added, add the broccoli and sweetcorn, and cook for 5 minutes, until the broccoli is just cooked. Add the mangetout and the lemon zest and juice, and cook for a further minute. Serve hot.

OMEGA-3 IS THE MAGIC NUMBER

Omega-3 has a number of health benefits including helping to improve eye, heart, joints and brain health, as well as fighting inflammation and depression. Most people get this nutrient from fatty acids in fish, but vegans may need to work harder to keep up their omega-3 levels. Snack on walnuts or edamame, add chia or hemp seeds to salads and smoothies or dress your meals with rapeseed oil.

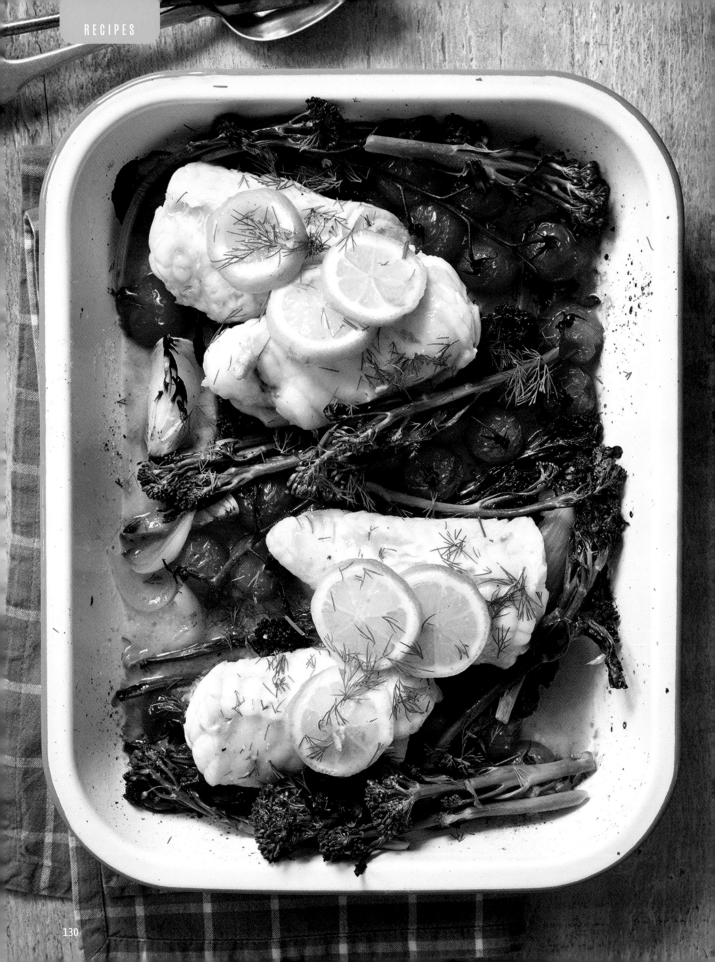

FISH & BROCCOLI TRAY BAKE

Monkfish is full of flavour and texture, making it a perfect combination with the nutrient-rich vegetables in this dish

SERVES **4** - READY IN **40** MINS

DF GF

Ingredients

- **1** onion, sliced into thin wedges
- **300 g** | **10 oz** cherry tomatoes, on the vine
- **200 g** | **7 oz** tenderstem broccoli
- **5 tbsp** good quality olive oil
- **4 x 150g** | **6 oz** pieces of monkfish fillet, chopped
- **1** lemon, sliced
- Olive oil, for drizzling
- **1** small bunch of dill, roughly chopped

Method

1. Heat the oven to 200C / Gas 6 / 400F. On a large roasting tray, toss the onion, tomatoes and broccoli together with the olive oil. Bake for 20 mins until cooked through and slightly charred.

2. Place the fish on top of the veg and add the lemon slices and a little drizzle of oil.

3. Return to the oven for 15 mins until just cooked through. Remove and serve, topped with chopped dill.

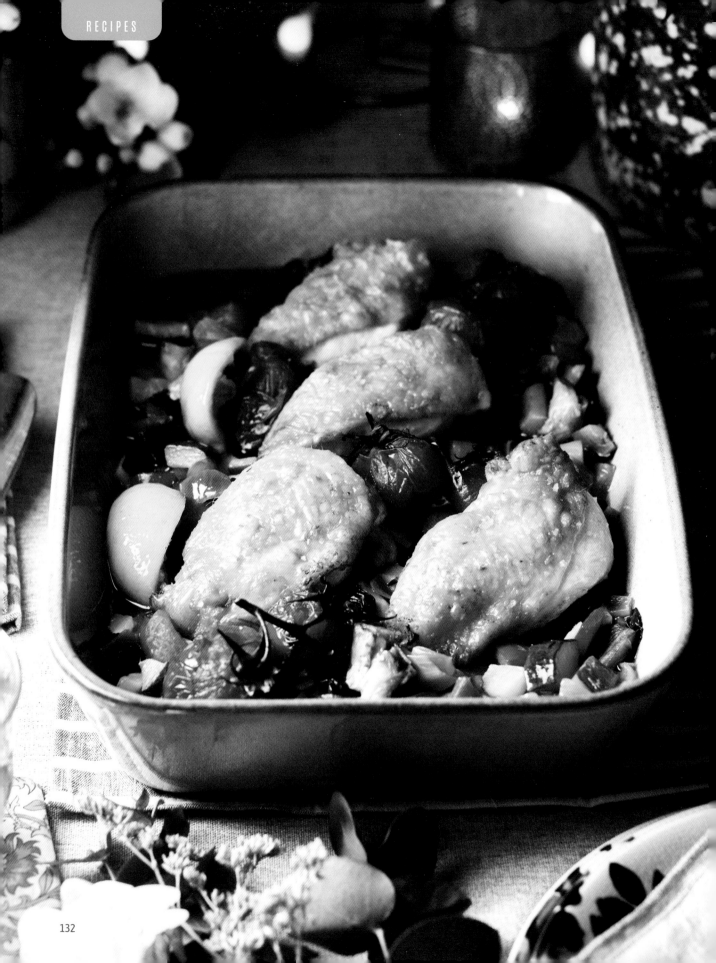

RATATOUILLE CHICKEN

Create a vibrant summery dish with this easy one-pot supper

SERVES 4 - READY IN 45 MINS   DF GF

Ingredients

- **1** large aubergine (eggplant), chopped into chunks
- **2** courgettes (zucchini), halved lengthways, deseeded and chopped
- **2** red onions, chopped
- **1** red (bell) pepper, chopped
- **1** yellow (bell) pepper, chopped
- **Small handful** of pitted green olives
- **4** garlic cloves, bashed
- **4 tbsp** extra virgin olive oil
- **Small bunch** of basil, leaves only
- **Few sprigs** of thyme, leaves picked
- **250 g | 9 oz** cherry tomatoes, on the vine
- **1** lemon
- **4** chicken breasts, skin on

Method

1. Heat the oven to 200C / Gas 6 / 400F. Mix together the aubergine, courgettes, red onions, peppers, olives and garlic in the roasting tin, drizzle over 2tbsp of the olive oil and mix with your hands. Tuck in the basil leaves and scatter over the thyme leaves.

2. Place the cherry tomatoes on top of the vegetables, quarter the lemon, squeeze the juice over the vegetables and tuck the squeezed quarters in the vegetable mix.

3. Rub the chicken breasts with the remaining 2tbsp olive oil and place skin side up on top of the vegetables. Season all over with salt and pepper. Roast in the oven for 30-35 mins until the chicken breasts are completely cooked through.

TIP

Replace the chicken with halloumi – pop onto the veg for the last 15 mins of cooking

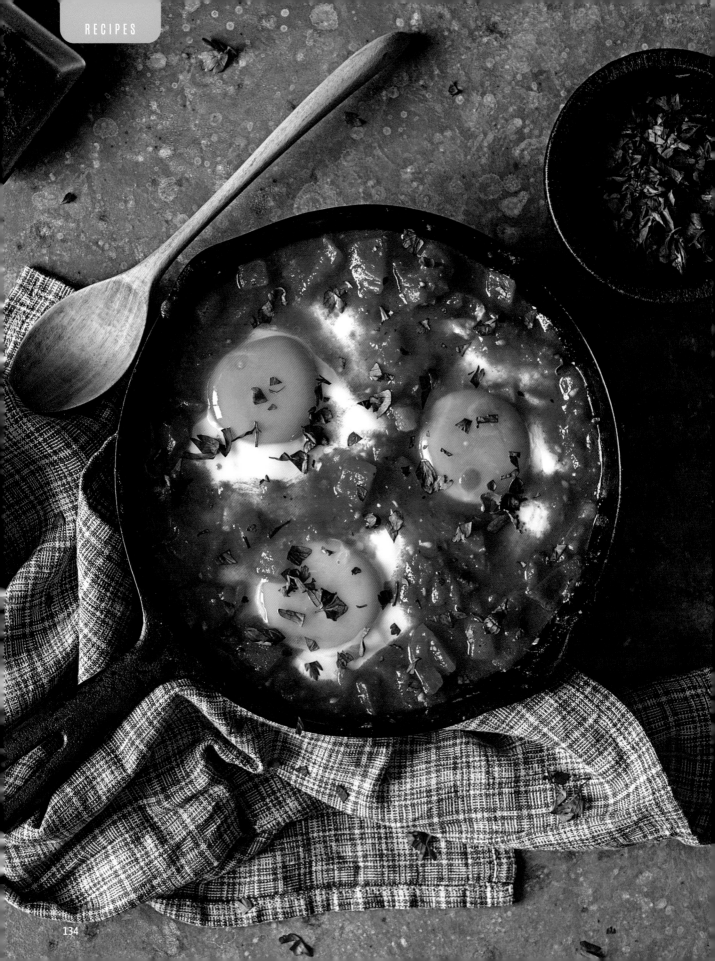

SHAKSHUKA

This spicy egg classic is always a popular brunch choice

SERVES **2** - READY IN **30** MINS

Ingredients

- **1** tbsp olive oil
- **2** onions chopped
- **1** red chilli, deseeded and finely chopped
- **1** garlic clove, sliced
- Small bunch of coriander, roughly chopped
- **2** cans | **400g** | **14oz** cherry tomatoes
- **1** tsp caster sugar
- **3-4** eggs
- **100g** | **3½oz** spinach
- Pinch Maldon sea salt

Method

1. Heat the oil in a frying pan that has a lid, soften the onions, chilli, garlic and coriander for 5 mins until soft.

2. Stir in the tomatoes and sugar, then bubble for 8-10 mins until thick. Stir in the spinach and coriander and cook for another minute.

3. Using the back of a large spoon, make wells in the sauce, then crack an egg into each one. Put a lid on the pan, then cook over a low heat for 6-8 mins, until the eggs are done to your liking.

4. Add a pinch of Maldon salt and serve with crusty bread.

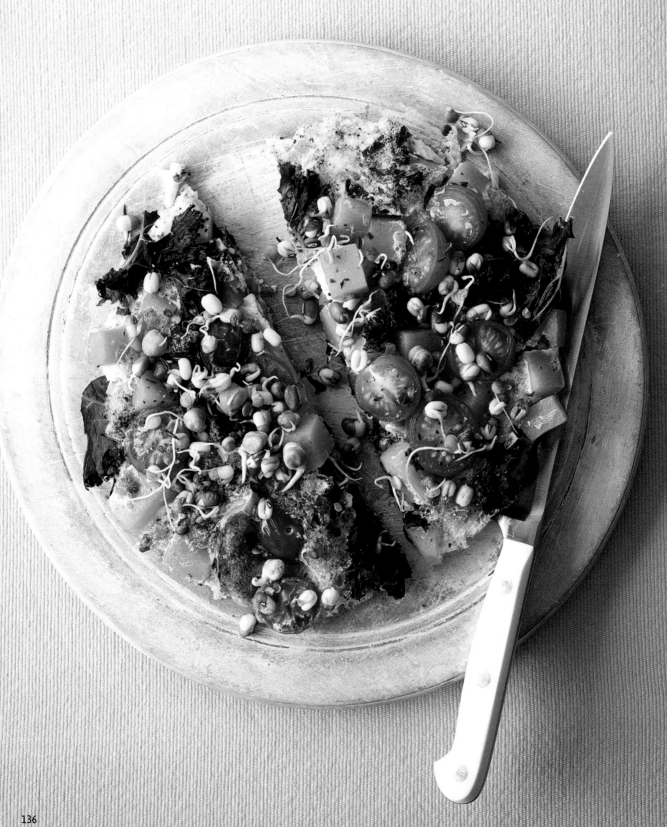

BUTTERNUT & KALE BREAKFAST STRATA

A healthy and filling breakfast for busy days

SERVES 2 - READY IN 20 MINS

DF

Ingredients

- **250g** | **8.8oz** peeled and seeded butternut squash, diced into approximately **1cm** | **½in** cubes
- **30g** | **1oz** roughly chopped curly kale leaves
- **120ml** | **4fl oz** liquid egg white or **4** free-range egg whites
- **¼ tsp** chilli flakes
- **2** sage leaves, finely chopped
- Salt and pepper
- **1** tbsp olive oil
- **6** baby cherry tomatoes, cut in half
- **20g** | **0.7oz** sprouting seeds, like Good4U Super Sprouts mix

Method

1. Put the diced squash in a vegetable steamer placed over a pan of barely boiling water, then cover and steam for 5 mins. Add the kale leaves and steam for a further 5-8 mins, or until both the squash and kale are just tender.

2. Whisk the egg white lightly with the chilli flakes, chopped sage leaves and a pinch of salt and pepper. Add oil into a non-stick frying pan with oil, then place over a medium heat and tip the squash and kale into the pan. Pour over the egg-white mixture and shake the pan gently to combine.

3. Scatter the cherry tomatoes over the top, then cook over a low heat for 3-5 mins, until just set. Remove from the heat, slide on to a plate and serve immediately, garnished with a handful of sprouting seeds.

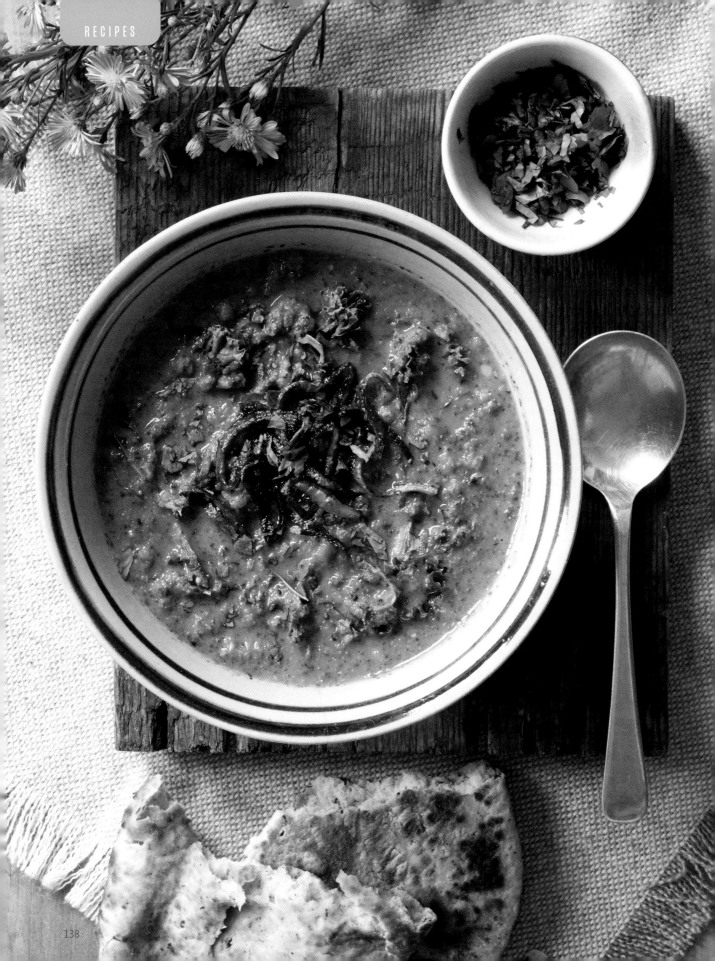

SPICED LENTIL SOUP

Comforting, creamy and packed full of goodness

SERVES 4 - READY IN 40 MINS

DF VE

Ingredients

- **2** tbsp olive oil, plus extra
- ½ tbsp garam masala
- Pinch of turmeric
- **1** tbsp black mustard seeds
- **2** onions, **1** diced and
  1 sliced into half moons
- **1** garlic clove, crushed
- **1** large carrot, diced
- **2** celery sticks, diced
- **200g** | **7oz** canned tomatoes
- **200ml** | **7fl oz** coconut milk
- **160g** | **5½oz** kale, shredded
- **400g** | **7oz** can green lentils
  in water, drained
- **30g** | **1oz** coriander,
  roughly chopped
- Mini naan bread,
  to serve, optional

Method

1. Heat the olive oil in a large pot, add the spices and mustard seeds. Once the mustard seeds begin to pop, add the diced onion, garlic, carrot and the celery. Cook for 10 mins or until the veg is softened.

2. Add the tomatoes, coconut milk, half the kale and 60ml (2fl oz) water. With a hand blender, blitz until smooth.

3. Stir in the rest of the kale and the lentils, and season to taste. Warm the soup through.

4. Heat the extra oil in a frying pan and fry the sliced onions until crisp. Then drain on kitchen towel.

5. To serve, top the soup with fried onions and coriander, and enjoy with mini naan bread, if liked.

TIP

If reheating leftover soup, add a little water to adjust the consistency.

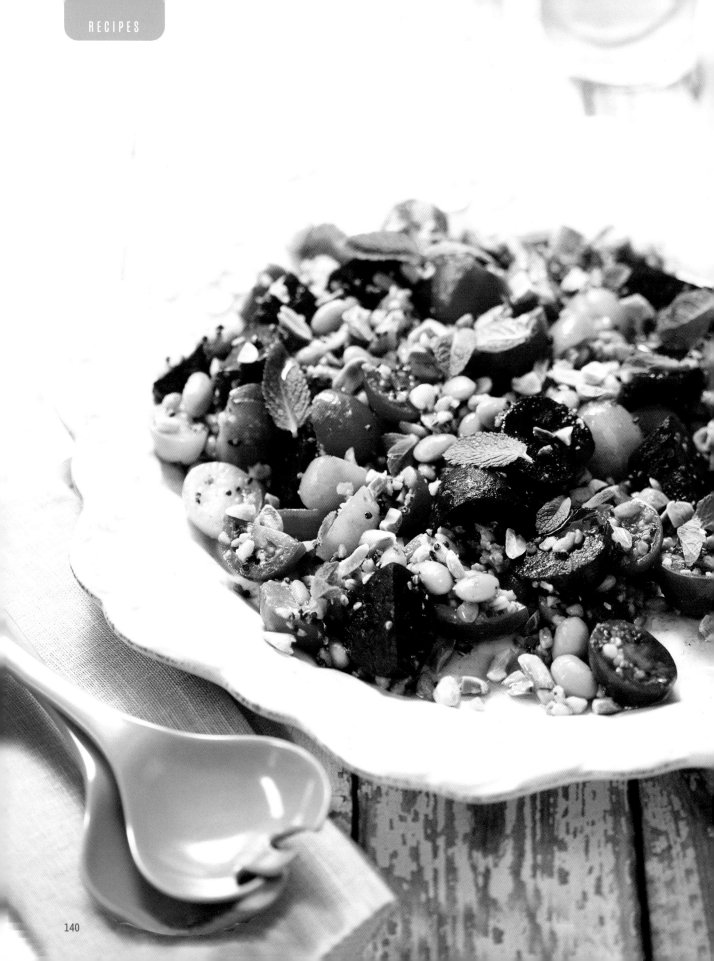

VEGGIE BOOST GRAIN SALAD

A diet rich in fibrous 'roughage' is good for your gut, so introducing beans, pulses and a variety of vegetables is a great way to start

SERVES **4** - READY IN **20** MINS

DF VE

Ingredients

- **150g** | **5oz** edamame (soya) beans
- **250g** | **9oz** cooked, mixed grains (e.g Merchant Gourmet Quinoa, lentils and wheatberries)
- **250g** | **9oz** tomatoes, cut in slices
- **250g** | **9oz** cooked baby beetroot, cut into wedges
- **25g** | **1oz** toasted peanuts, chopped
- Fresh mint, to serve

For the dressing

- **1 tbsp** sesame oil
- **1 tbsp** olive oil
- **1 tsp** rice vinegar
- **1 tsp** soy sauce

Method

1. Blanch edamame beans in boiling water for 2 mins, refresh under cold running water. Put grains in a large bowl. Mix the dressing ingredients and stir through the grains.

2. Add the remaining ingredients and serve.

TIP

Feel free to serve it as a side dish to go with grilled fish, chicken or lamb.

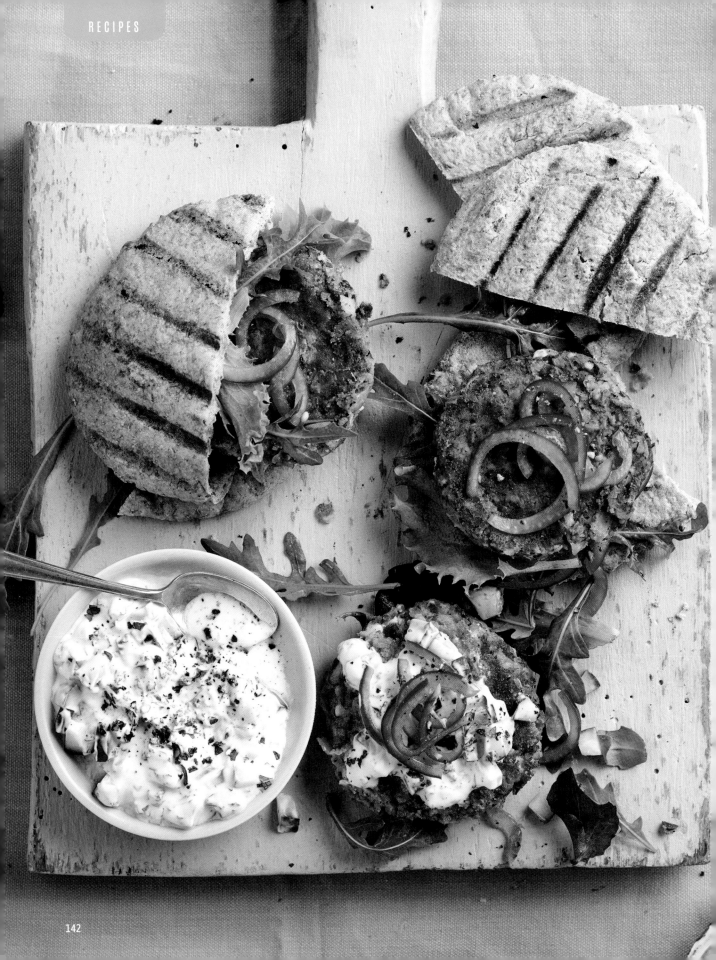

GREEK-INSPIRED BEAN BURGERS

These burgers are a great meat-free option for lunch or dinner!

SERVES 2 - READY IN 20 MINS

Ingredients

- **1 tbsp** red wine vinegar
- **75g | 2½oz** 0% fat Greek style natural yogurt or vegan alternative
- **2 tbsp** roughly chopped fresh mint
- ½ cucumber, finely diced
- **2** wholemeal pitta breads, halved
- Bag mixed salad leaves, to serve

For the burgers

- **1½** tbsp olive oil
- **1** red onion, ½ diced and ½ finely sliced
- **1** garlic clove, crushed
- **400g | 14oz** tin mixed beans, drained and rinsed
- **30g | 1oz** fresh wholemeal breadcrumbs
- **1 tbsp** dried oregano
- **1 tsp** chilli flakes
- **½ tsp** dried mint
- Zest and juice of ½ lemon
- **75g | 2½oz** reduced-fat Greek-style salad cheese or vegan alternative

Method

1. For the burgers, heat ½ tbsp of the oil in a frying pan and cook the diced onion and the garlic until soft. Add the mixed beans to the pan to warm through. Use a potato masher to crush them into a paste. Mix in the breadcrumbs, oregano, chilli flakes, mint, lemon zest and juice, and cheese. Press and shape into 4 patties.

2. Pour the vinegar over the sliced onion. Mix together and set aside.

3. Heat the remaining 1 tbsp oil in the frying pan and cook the burgers for 4 mins on each side until cooked through.

4. Meanwhile, mix the yogurt, mint and cucumber. Toast the pitta breads and open up the pockets. Top the bean burgers with some of the sliced onion. Serve with the salad leaves, the pittas and the refreshing minty yoghurt.

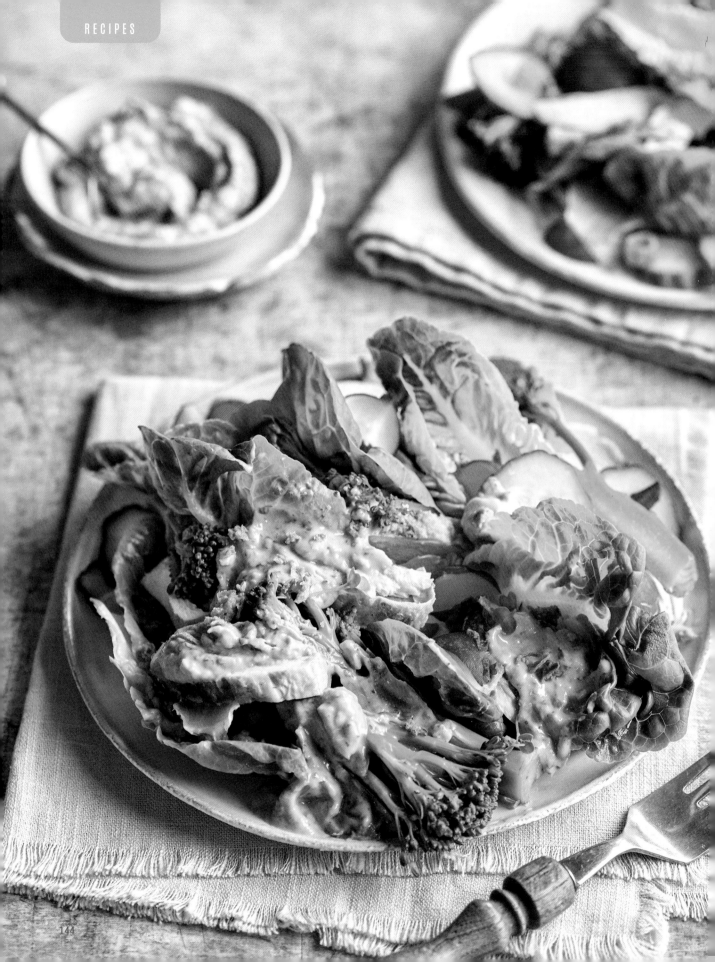

GREEN GODDESS CHICKEN SALAD

The avocado in the dressing creates a thick sauce that reminds us of Caesar salad

SERVES **2** - READY IN **10** MINS

GF

Ingredients

- **150g** | **5oz** Tenderstem broccoli
- **2** Little Gem lettuce, leaves separated
- **6cm** | **2½in** piece cucumber, thinly sliced
- **6** radishes, thinly sliced
- **150g** | **5oz** leftover roast chicken, shredded, any skin removed
- **4** salad onions, thinly sliced
- **½** tbsp crispy onions
- Salad cress

For the dressing

- **1** baby avocado, stoned and diced
- **1** small garlic clove
- **4** tbsp 0% fat Greek-style natural yoghurt
- Zest and juice of ½ lemon
- **1** tbsp roughly chopped fresh tarragon or coriander

Method

1. For the dressing, whizz all the ingredients in a blender until smooth. Check the seasoning and add a splash of water if it's a little thick.

2. Blanch the broccoli in a pan of boiling, lightly salted water for 3-4 mins until tender. Drain and cool under running water.

3. Arrange the lettuce, cucumber, radishes, broccoli, chicken and salad onions onto 2 serving plates. Drizzle over the dressing, then scatter with crispy onions and salad cress.

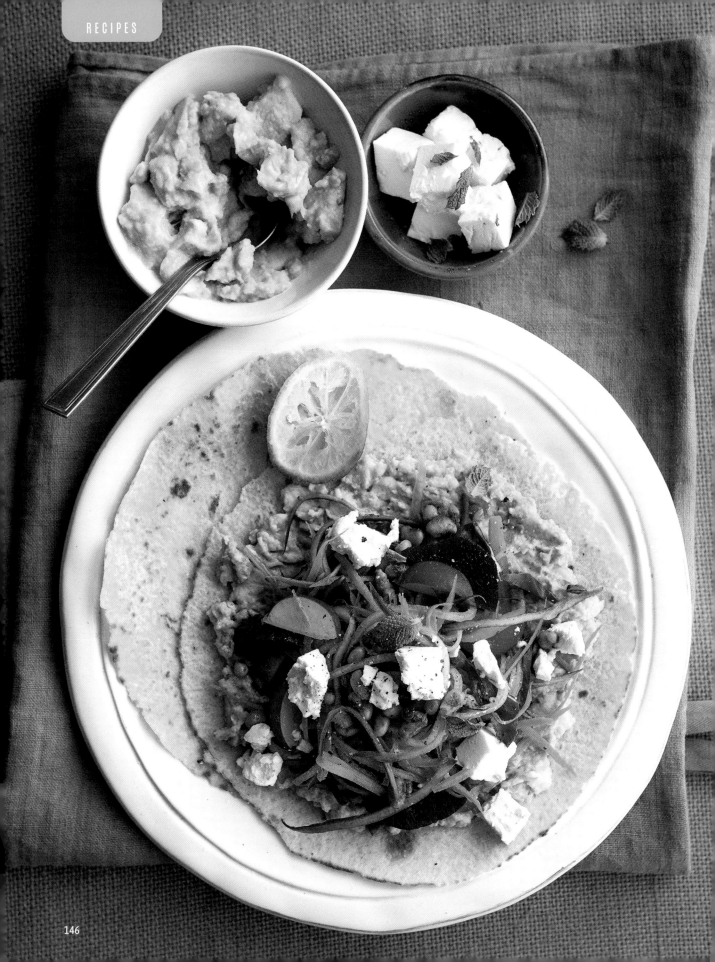

PERI-PERI RAINBOW WRAP

Bursting with colourful veg, this healthy meal is quick to make

SERVES **2** - READY IN **25** MINS

Ingredients

- Olive oil spray
- **400g** | **14oz** can black-eyed beans, drained and rinsed
- **1 tsp** peri-peri seasoning
- **1** avocado, stoned, peeled and chopped
- Juice of ½ lime
- **2** wholemeal or corn tortilla wraps
- **150g** | **5.3oz** red cabbage, shredded
- **1** large carrot, grated
- ⅓ cucumber, cut into julienne strips
- **4** radishes, quartered
- **100g** | **3.5oz** feta
- Few sprigs of mint
- **75g** | **2.6oz** beetroot, cut in wedges

Method

1. Spray a non-stick pan with oil and gently fry the beans and peri-peri seasoning for 10 mins until crispy.

2. In a bowl, mash the avocado with the lime juice.

3. Warm the wraps according to pack instructions and spread with avocado.

4. Combine cabbage, carrot, cucumber and radishes, then stir in the beans. Pile on top of the tortillas, sprinkle over the feta, mint and beetroot to serve.

TIP

To make this vegan, replace the feta with vegan cheese.

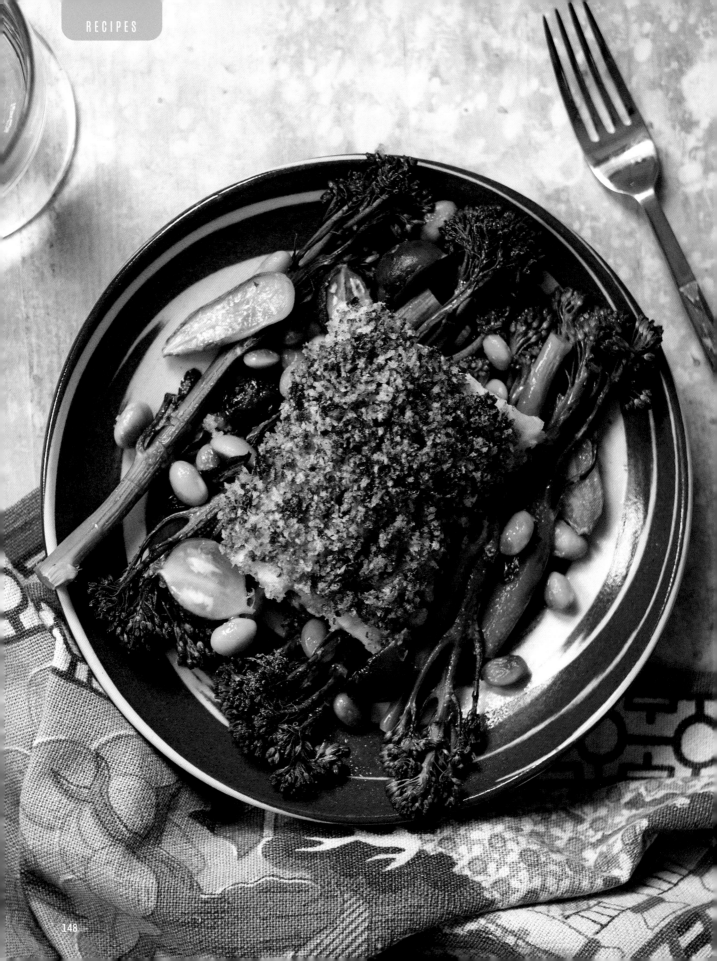

MISO COD WITH TENDERSTEM BROCCOLI

Not only is broccoli tasty and vibrant, it's great for the gut and supports immunity

SERVES **2** - READY IN **35** MINS   DF

Ingredients

- **30g** | **1oz** panko breadcrumbs
- **1 tsp** brown rice miso
- **1 tbsp** olive oil
- **Small handful** chopped fresh coriander
- **2** pieces of cod loin
- **200g** | **7oz** Tenderstem broccoli
- **100g** | **3.5oz** edamame beans
- **8-10** radishes, cut in half
- Miso soup sachet – we used Itsu
- **1 tbsp** rice wine vinegar
- **1 tsp** sesame oil
- **1 tsp** honey
- **½ tsp** light soy sauce

Method

1. Heat the oven to 200°C / 390°F / Gas 6. Mix the breadcrumbs with the miso, oil and coriander. Coat the top of each cod loin with the panko mixture and set aside.

2. Layer the bottom of a deep roasting tin with the broccoli, beans and radishes.

3. Mix the miso soup sachet with 200ml boiling water, rice wine vinegar, sesame oil, honey and soy sauce. Pour over the veg and roast for 5 mins. Remove from the oven and place the cod on top. Bake for a further 20 mins.

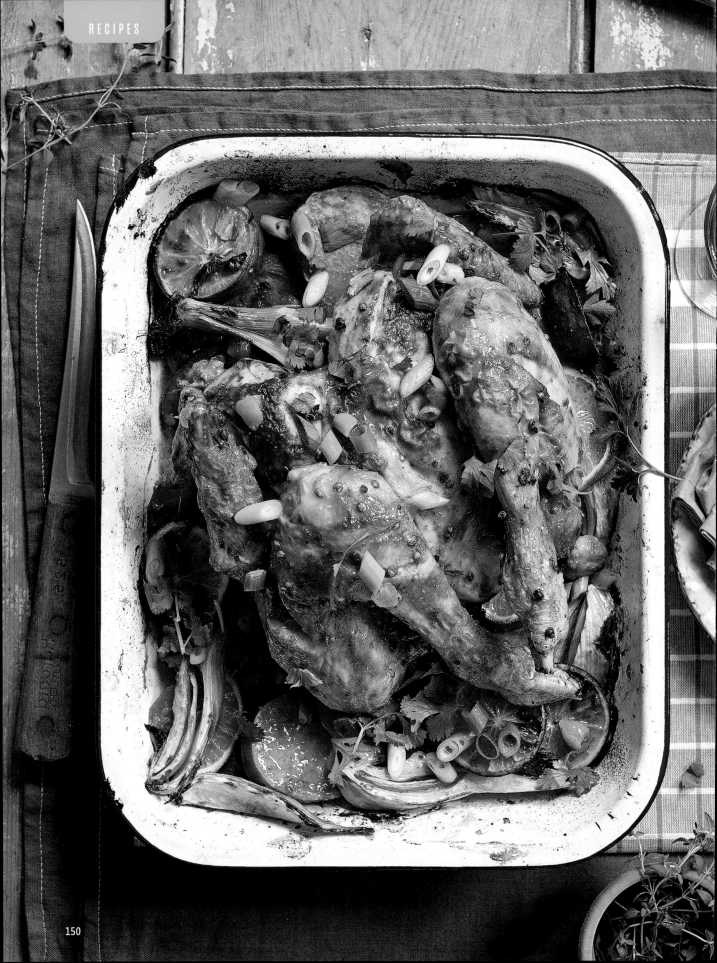

TURMERIC ROAST CHICKEN WITH ORANGE & FENNEL

A comforting one-pot dish that will help you to beat inflammation

SERVES **4** - READY IN **1** HR **30** MINS   DF

Ingredients

- **1** whole free-range chicken, spatchcocked
- **125ml** | **5fl oz** olive oil
- **2** garlic cloves
- **1 tbsp** coriander seeds
- **1 tsp** dried turmeric or 1 tbsp peeled and finely grated fresh turmeric
- **4** medium sweet potatoes, sliced into rounds
- **80g** | **3oz** dried apricots, roughly chopped
- **1** orange, thickly sliced
- **1 bulb** fennel, cut into chunks
- **1 glass** of white wine
- **1 bunch** of parsley, roughly chopped
- **4** spring onions, sliced

Method

1. Blitz the olive oil, garlic, coriander seeds and turmeric together in a small processor. Score the chicken skin a few times, then rub with the marinade. Cover and chill for at least 1 hour or overnight.

2. Heat the oven to 180°C Fan / 200°C/ 400°F /Gas 6. Put the potatoes, apricots, orange slices and fennel in a large roasting tin. Then put the marinated chicken on top, skin side up, and pour over the wine along with as any leftover marinade. Season well and cover with foil.

3. Roast for 30 mins. Remove the foil and reduce the heat to 160°C Fan / 180°C / 350°F/Gas 4. Roast for another 45 mins, until the chicken is cooked through and golden. Garnish with parsley and spring onions to serve.

TIP

Thanks to its high levels of curcumin, turmeric has powerful antioxidant and anti-inflammatory qualities.

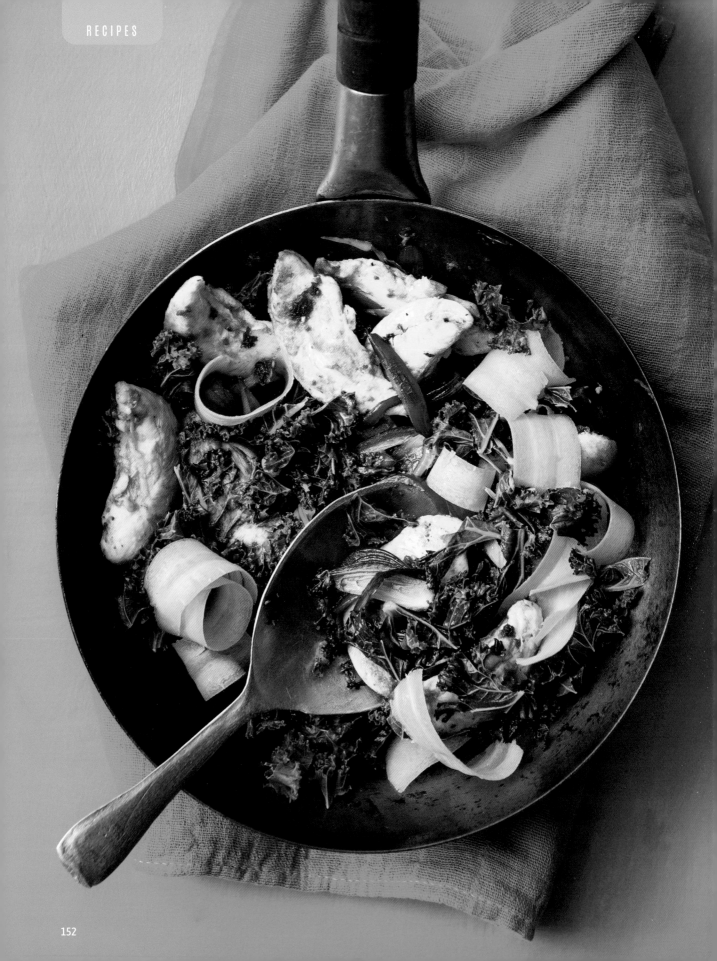

CHICKEN &
KALE STIR FRY

This flavourful and simple meal contains anti-inflammatory turmeric and miso

SERVES 4 - READY IN 25 MINS

DF

Ingredients

- **425g** | **15oz** mini chicken breast fillets, or regular sized fillets sliced into smaller pieces
- **2.5cm** | **1in** root ginger, peeled, grated
- **2** garlic cloves, grated
- **1** lemon, grated zest and juice
- **2 tbsp** rapeseed oil
- **¼ tsp** turmeric
- **2** red onions, sliced
- **250g** | **8.8oz** curly kale, chopped
- **1 tbsp** miso paste
- **2** carrots, peeled

Method

1. Put chicken into a shallow dish and season. Sprinkle over ginger, garlic and lemon zest. Squeeze on the lemon juice and stir to mix evenly.

2. Heat oil in a wok and fry the chicken for 3 mins without stirring. Sprinkle with the turmeric, turn and cook for 3 more mins.

3. Push the chicken to the side and add onions. Cook for 3 mins. Add the kale. Stir miso into 200ml | 7fl oz boiling water, cook for 3 mins.

4. Use a peeler on the carrots to create ribbons. Add to the wok for 2 mins. Serve with quinoa.

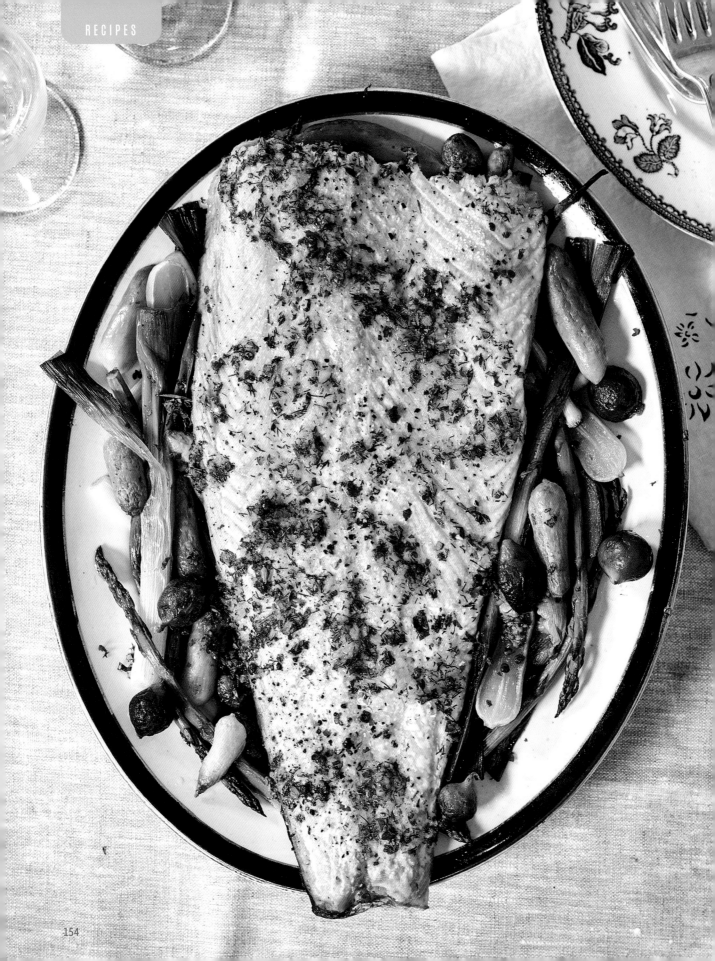

ROAST SIDE OF SALMON WITH BLUSHING VEG

This mouthwatering salmon is so easy to prepare and will make a delightful, impressive centrepiece at your table

SERVES 8 - READY IN 40 MINS

Ingredients

- **450g** | **1lb** mixed radishes
- **250g** | **8¾oz** asparagus tips
- **300g** | **10½oz** baby leeks
- **3 tbsp** olive oil
- Zest of **1** lemon
- **1kg** | **2lb 3¼oz** side salmon, skin on

For the Dressing

- **1** banana shallot, finely chopped
- **Large bunch** of fresh herbs (we used parsley, dill and lemon thyme)
- **50g** | **1¾oz** olive oil
- Juice of **1** lemon
- **1 tsp** cracked pink peppercorns, to garnish

Method

1. Heat the oven to 200°C / 400°F / Gas 6. Place the radishes, asparagus and baby leeks on a large baking tray, and drizzle with 2tbsp of the oil, and season with salt and pepper. Toss everything together with the lemon zest to coat the vegetables evenly.

2. On a separate baking tray lined with parchment, place the salmon on top, skin-side down, and brush with the remaining olive oil. Season well.

3. Place both trays in the oven for 25 minutes, until the salmon is just cooked through and the vegetables are nicely roasted. Serve hot or at room temperature with the dressing.

4. For the dressing, simply blitz all the ingredients together, and drizzle over the salmon and vegetables.

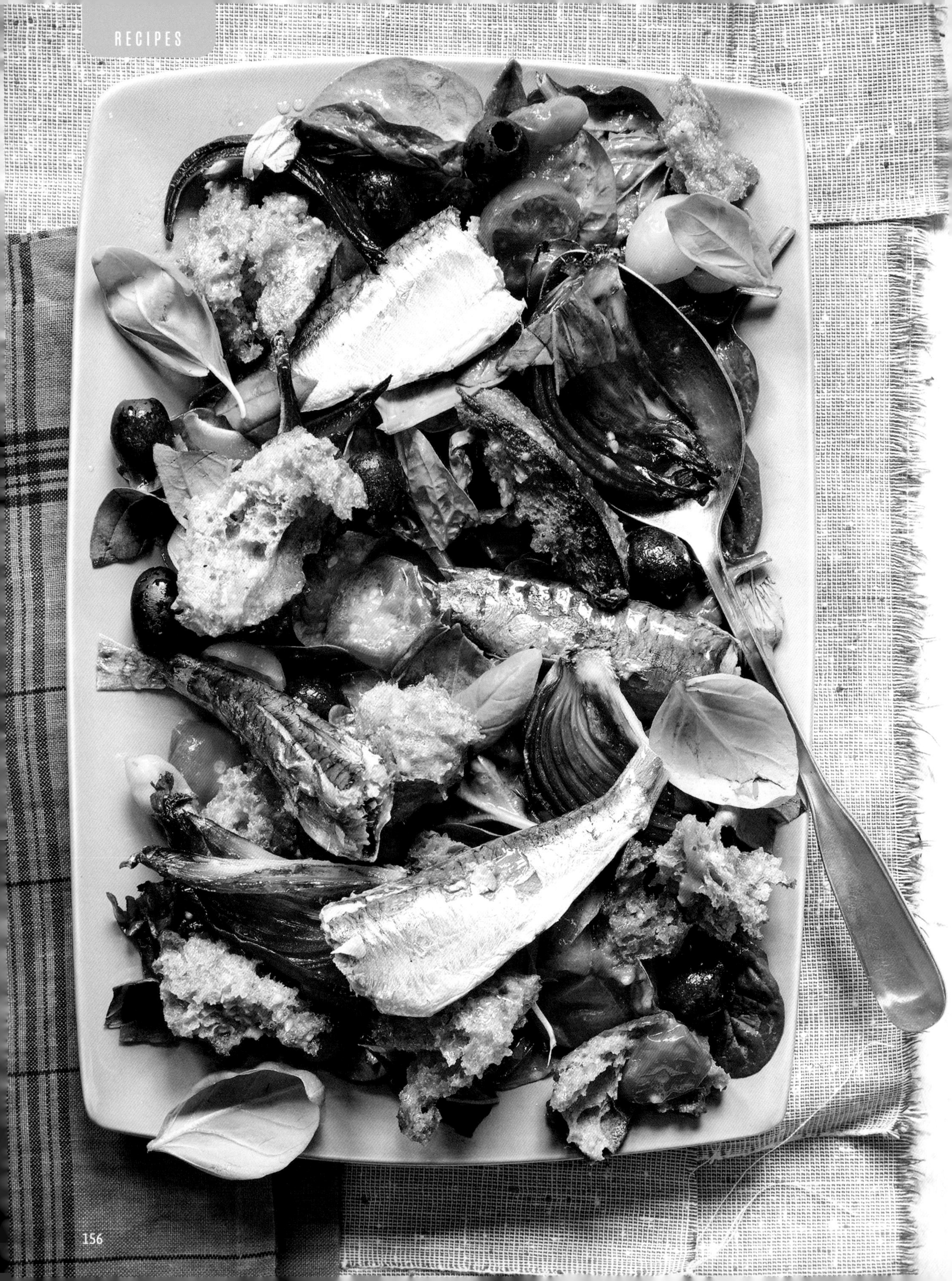

SARDINE & SPINACH PANZANELLA

A hearty salad that is packed full of flavour and nutrition

SERVES 4 - READY IN 35 MINS

Ingredients

- 1 red onion, cut into wedges
- 2 tbsp olive oil
- 250g | 9oz tomatoes, halved
- 150g | 5oz wholemeal bread, roughly torn into chunks
- 1 garlic clove, crushed
- Thin strips of rind from ½ lemon
- 2 x 120g | 4½oz cans sardines
- 75g | 3oz spinach leaves
- 45g | 1½oz black olives
- 30g | 1oz basil leaves, torn

For the Dressing

- 1 garlic clove, crushed
- 125ml | 4½fl oz olive oil
- 3 tbsp white wine vinegar
- 1 tsp Dijon mustard

Method

1. Heat the oven to 180°C / 350°F / Gas 4. Place the onion wedges on a baking tray, drizzle with 1tbsp olive oil and roast for 15 mins. Add the tomatoes and roast for 10 mins.

2. Put the bread on a separate baking tray, drizzle with 1tbsp oil, scatter over the garlic and lemon rind and roast for 10 mins.

3. Combine all the dressing ingredients, stir in the roasted tomatoes and season to taste. Mix together the onion, bread, sardines, spinach, olives and basil on a platter and pour over the tomato dressing to serve.

TIP

Sardines are a nutritional bargain – rich in fatty acids, protein and calcium.

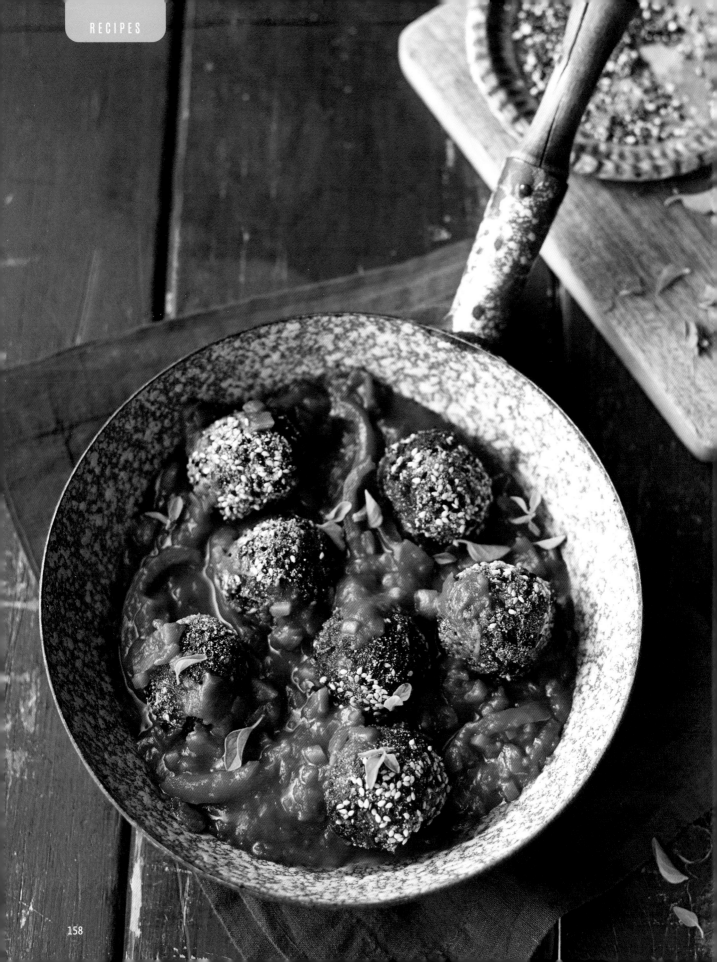

BEETROOT BALLS IN A SPANISH-STYLE SAUCE

Meatless meatballs doesn't mean flavourless with these balls!

SERVES 4 - READY IN 50 MINS

DF

Ingredients

- **400g** | **14.1oz** raw beetroot, trimmed and peeled
- **400g** | **14.1oz** sweet or waxy potatoes
- **400g** | **14.1oz** can chickpeas, drained, rinsed and dried
- **3** garlic cloves, crushed
- A good pinch of chilli powder
- **2 tbsp** polenta
- **1 tbsp** sesame seeds
- **3 tbsp** sunflower oil
- **1** onion, thinly sliced
- **1** small carrot, finely chopped
- **1** red pepper, deseeded and thinly sliced
- **2 x 200g** | **7oz** cartons passata
- **200ml** | **6.8fl oz** veg stock
- **¾ tsp** sweet smoked paprika
- **Small handful** of oregano leaves

Method

1. Wearing clean rubber gloves, coarsely grate the beetroot, then squeeze out the excess water with your hands.

2. Pierce the potatoes all over, then cook in the microwave on High for 6 mins, or until cooked through. Leave to cool.

3. Put the chickpeas in a mixing bowl and roughly break up with the back of a fork. Scoop out potato flesh and add to the mix, along with the beetroot, garlic and chilli powder. Mix well with your hands, then shape into 16 balls.

4. Mix the polenta and sesame seeds together, then roll the balls in this mixture, one at a time, and cover loosely with foil. Leave to firm up in the fridge for around 1 hr (or more if you like).

5. Heat 1 tbsp of the oil in a pan over a medium heat, add the onion and cook for 4 mins, or until softened and browning. Add the carrot and red pepper, mix and cook for 2 mins more. Add the passata, stock, a pinch of sugar and the paprika. Bring to the boil, cover and simmer for 25 mins.

6. Heat the rest of the oil in a frying pan over a medium heat. Brown the beetroot balls, in batches, on all sides. Add to the sauce with the oregano.

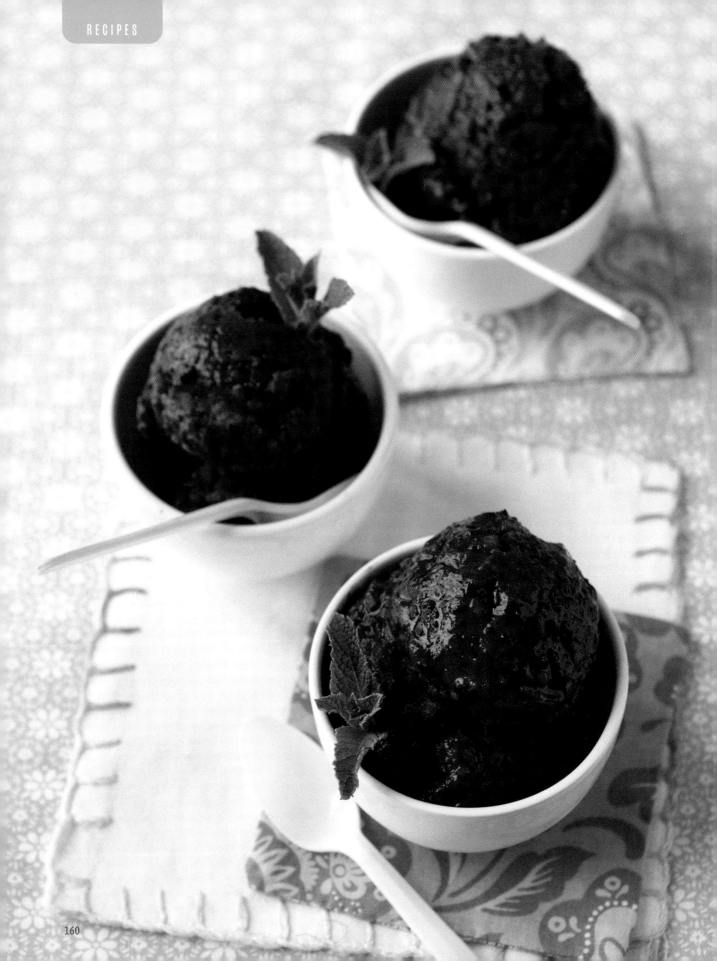

QUICK BERRY & WATERMELON SORBET

The perfect treat to have stored in your freezer

SERVES **4-5** - READY IN **10** MINS PLUS CHILLING TIME

DF GF VE

Ingredients

- **450 g** | **16 oz** | **3 cups** frozen berries
- **175 g** | **6 oz 1** | **1 cup** prepared watermelon chunks, frozen
- Juice of **1** lemon
- **2** tbsp icing sugar
- Mint leaves, for garnish

Method

1. Remove the frozen fruits from the freezer and leave them until they just start to soften slightly. Tip them into a blender, along with the lemon juice and sugar, and then purée until smooth.

2. If the mixture is very soft, return it to the freezer until it's firm enough to scoop into balls. Serve sorbet garnished with mint.

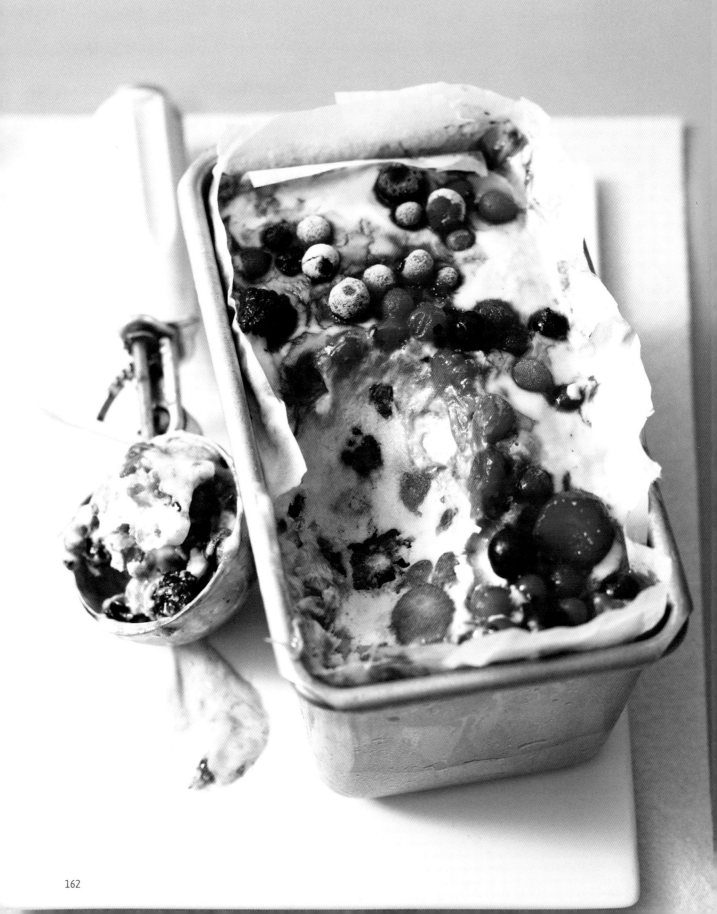

BERRY FROZEN YOGURT

This easy dessert is so quick to put together and works well as a treat

SERVES 8 - READY IN 10 MINS PLUS FREEZING

Ingredients

- **250ml** | **9oz** | **1** can coconut cream
- **375ml** | **12¾fl oz** coconut milk yogurt
- **3 tbsp** icing sugar or sweetener
- **300g** | **10½oz** mixed frozen berries

Method

1. Whisk the coconut cream, yogurt and icing sugar together until smooth. Stir in the berries and crush slightly. Turn into a container and freeze until firm, preferably overnight.

2. Allow to soften at room temperature for half an hour before serving.

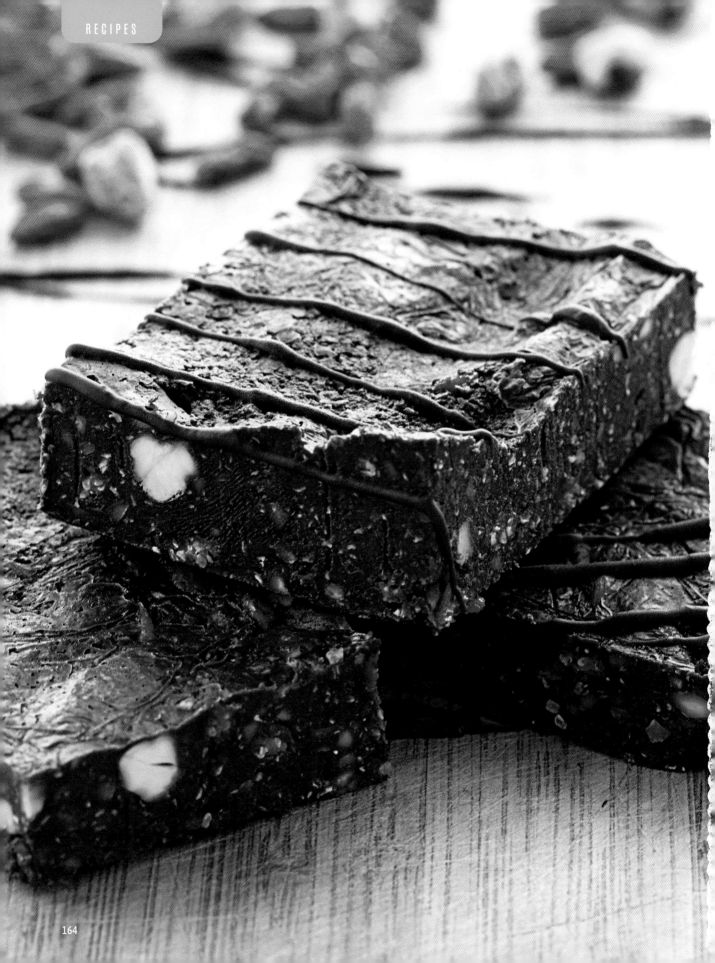

RAW CHOCOLATE BROWNIE

These no-bake fudgy brownies are the perfect sweet treat

SERVES 4 - READY IN 10 MINS

VE

Ingredients

- **450g** | **16oz** | **3** cups Medjool dates, pitted
- **220g** | **7¾oz** | **1½** cups blanched hazelnuts
- **6 tbsp** cacao powder
- **2 tbsp** date syrup (or maple syrup)
- **110g** | **4oz** | **1** cup goji berries, roughly chopped
- **125g** | **4¼oz** | ½ cup crushed pistachio nuts
- **100g** | **3½oz** vegan dark chocolate
- Pinch sea salt, to garnish

Method

1. Toast the hazelnuts in a dry pan over a medium-high heat (alternatively, roast them in a hot oven) for about 5 minutes or until golden and fragrant. Set aside to cool.

2. Once the hazelnuts are cooled, blitz them in a food processor until they form a crumbly sand-like mixture.

3. Add the dates and blend again before adding the cacao and date syrup. Blend further until everything is mixed together.

4. Pour the brownie mix into a large bowl, and mix in the chopped goji berries and crushed pistachios. Stir it together until everything is evenly distributed.

5. Press the mix into a baking tray and pop it in the fridge for 3-4 hours to set.

6. Once chilled, melt the chocolate and drizzle it over the top, chill again until the chocolate has set, then serve with a sprinkling of sea salt.

Image: Getty